Stepping into Palliative Care

A Handbook for Community Pro

Edited by

Jo C

Forewords by
Professor Philip Burnard
Vice Dean of Nursing Studies
University of Wales College of Medicine
and
Dr Robert S Martin
Medical Director
Palliative Care Unit
Hartford Hospital, USA

5

Radcliffe Medical Press

© 2000 Jo Cooper

Radcliffe Medical Press Ltd
18 Marcham Road, Abingdon, Oxon OX14 1AA

British Library Cataloguing in Publication Data

A catalogue record for this book is available from the British Library.

ISBN 1 85775 303 8

Typeset by Acorn Bookwork, Salisbury, Wiltshire
Printed and bound by TJ International Ltd, Padstow, Cornwall

Contents

Forewords   v

Preface   ix

List of contributors   xiii

Acknowledgements   xv

Part One: Practical approaches to individual care

1   Introduction to pain control   3
Trevor Mitten

2   Symptom control   23
Susanna Hill

3   Continuous subcutaneous infusion   55
Jo Cooper and Trevor Mitten

4   Mouthcare   67
Elizabeth Potter

5   Lymphoedema   81
Mary Woods

6   Wound care   89
Mark Collier

7   Terminal restlessness   105
Jo Cooper

Part Two: Practical approaches to the needs of the individual

8   Hearing the pain of the carer   119
Mandy Redgrove and Audrey Smyth

9   Spirituality: sharing the journey   127
Rosemary Booth

10   Bereavement   137
      Jenny Penson

Part Three: Working together to provide palliative care

11   Making the most of palliative care services
            Section 1: The role of the specialist nurse   151
            Francesca Thompson
            Section 2: The role of the hospice in-patient unit   161
            Suzanne Lesley Cockerton
            Section 3: The role of the hospice day unit   169
            Pearl McDaid

12   Integrated care pathways   179
      John E Ellershaw

Part Four: Working together and making it work

13   Communication   189
      David B Cooper

14   Stress issues in palliative care: caring for the community professional   197
      Robin J Davidson

15   Management issues in palliative care: caring for the community
      professional   207
      Suzanne Mace

Part Five: Special considerations

16   The special needs of the neurological patient   223
      David Oliver

17   Legal aspects of palliative care   235
      Bridgit Dimond

Appendix: Useful contacts   249

Index   255

Foreword

This is a refreshing book in all respects. First, it is clearly written by experts in the field. The writers of this book are all either practitioners or educators in this area. Secondly, the layout and presentation allow for easy reading and for the digestion of a great deal of information in a palatable format. Thirdly, although it is written for beginners in the field, it will act as a vital sourcebook of information and ideas for those already working in the area. Those reading it are likely to feel encouraged and refreshed by it.

Overall, the emphasis is practical. The first two sections focus on practical approaches to helping the individual. The second two sections explore working as a team or a group – essential in the field of palliative care, where so many individuals are both involved and affected. The final section offers two valuable chapters on the special needs of the neurological patient and on legal implications.

The structure of the book and the use of copious examples of good practice both ensure that what is offered is easily assimilated. The reader is also asked to identify his or her own baseline knowledge at the beginning of each chapter. This innovative idea is another example of how this book can both stimulate and educate.

This volume is going to be a resource of great value. It will help students of all kinds in the community care, medical, nursing, social work and psychological professions. It will also be of immeasurable use to those engaged in the practice of palliative care. Finally, it is a book to be used as a resource. All clinics, community-care centres, hospitals and hospices will want a copy in their libraries. The editor and the contributors are to be congratulated on having produced such a useful and usable text.

Professor Philip Burnard
Vice Dean of Nursing Studies
University of Wales College of Medicine
February 2000

Foreword

For many years hospice care was a narrowly defined and somewhat jealously guarded area of medical care, closely associated with cancer and death. On many occasions this association has resulted in late referrals and reluctance to accept hospice care by patients with diagnoses other than cancer.

More recently, the term *palliative care* has increasingly been used to describe the type of care most people want for their loved ones (or for themselves) at the end of life, or at any point in the trajectory of a potentially terminal illness.

This refreshing handbook is an excellent introduction to the 'nuts and bolts' of palliative care. Written with a minimum of medical jargon, it covers a wide array of problems and solutions commonly encountered by caregivers, and includes useful references and stimulating questions at the end of most chapters.

Stepping into Palliative Care should be a valuable tool for professionals who want to learn about this exciting and growing sub-speciality of medical care.

Robert S Martin MD, FACP
Medical Director
Palliative Care Unit
Hartford Hospital
Hartford
February 2000

Preface

Whilst prognosis is a consideration to the rehabilitation plan,
it should never be a contra-indication to the effort...

Gunn, 1984

Stepping into Palliative Care is primarily intended for those new to the field of palliative care and/or care professionals with some basic knowledge who wish to update themselves.

In order to meet the requirements of the individual who is exposed to palliative care provision, the community professional will need education and training targeted at the 'how to' element of professional practice and patient management. For the community professional who is in daily or occasional contact with the patient, their family and significant others affected by cancer it is an integral part of his or her professional daily life. For health and social care professionals to be able to identify problems, instigate interventions and support services, and actively monitor interventions, it is essential that there is a clear pathway of perception of the active role that each one of us plays, and participates in – be that before, during and/or after palliative care has been accessed.

This book is a practical, basic guide to the many and varied problems faced by the patient, their family and significant others. It asserts how the community nurse can influence the effective outcome of such interventions.

The book offers a first-step introduction, relevant to the needs of the community professional, in a clear, concise and understandable format. It is divided into five sections as follows.

- Part One: Practical approaches to individual care.
- Part Two: Practical approaches to the needs of the individual.
- Part Three: Working together to provide palliative care.
- Part Four: Working together and making it work.
- Part Five: Special considerations.

Each section builds on the last to offer an overview of the needs relating to the individual who encounters palliative care. Where applicable, a chapter makes full and effective use of 'at-a-glance' practical features including boxes, tables, figures, self-assessment questions and case studies. 'Suggested reading' sections point the reader in the direction of further knowledge and information. At the end of the book there is a helpful appendix of useful contacts that can provide more information, advice and guidance for the health and social care professional, the patient and their relative(s).

The book aims to address the difficulties associated with pain and symptom control. It looks at how we can identify the problems, and encourages the introduction of whatever intervention may be therapeutic. It is hoped that by advocating this basic, easy-to-use practical format it will facilitate the professional's ability to examine the guidance and make useful advances in the way in which they approach palliative care. It is hoped that the book will demonstrate to the health and social care professional that their efforts can and will affect their practice and how that impacts on the needs of the patient, their relative(s) and significant others.

Intended as a 'dip-in-and-out' resource, the book is aimed at the community health and social care professional who is new to palliative care. It will be of value to community nurses, health visitors, social workers, medical practitioners and medical trainees, those involved in spiritual and psychological care, as well as the individual practitioner wishing to update or refresh existing knowledge and expertise. It will also be relevant to those undertaking education and training for nurse registration.

This book is a starting point to further education and training. It attempts to provide some of the answers, discuss some of the issues surrounding palliative care, and direct the reader towards further development.

'I can't help thinking of Rembrant's paintings, where the light is so glorious
That it makes even the darkness look beautiful' – you could say that the
Light only looked so glorious because of the darkness around it

Kearney

Jo Cooper
February 2000

Cautionary note

Throughout this book, reference is made to drugs and dosages. The authors and editor have made every effort to check the accuracy of this information and to ensure that it is up to date. However, it is important to note that drugs, dosages and indications for use can change as current research and developments provide new supporting evidence. It is imperative that the drug, dosage and indications are checked by the prescribing individual, at the time when the medication is to be used, with the current recommendations. It is also advised that those administering the medication should check the evidence available at that time. The pharmacist is a valuable resource for all aspects of drug administration and prescribing information.

List of contributors

Rosemary Booth
Clinical Nurse Specialist
North Devon Hospice
Barnstaple

Suzanne Lesley Cockerton
Director of Patient Care
St Elizabeth Hospice
Ipswich

Mark Collier
Nurse Consultant/Senior Lecturer
CRICP Thames Valley University

David B Cooper
Freelance author
Editor, *Service Development*

Jo Cooper
Macmillan Clinical Nurse Specialist
North Devon Hospice
Barnstaple

Robin J Davidson
Consultant Clinical Psychologist
Belvoir Park Hospital
Belfast

Bridgit Dimond
Emeritus Professor
University of Glamorgan
Pontypridd

John E Ellershaw
Medical Director/Consultant in Palliative
  Medicine
Marie Curie Centre
Liverpool

Susanna Hill
Associate Specialist in Palliative Care
North Devon Hospice
Barnstaple

Pearl McDaid
Day Hospital Systems Coordinator
Peace Hospital
Watford

Suzanne Mace
Patient Services Manager
North Devon Hospice
Barnstaple

Trevor Mitten
Clinical Nurse Specialist
North Devon Hospice
Barnstaple

David Oliver
Medical Director and Consultant in
  Palliative Medicine
Wisdom Hospice
Rochester

Jenny Penson
Education Manager
North Devon Hospice
Barnstaple

Elizabeth Potter
Macmillan Head & Neck Specialist Nurse
Southmead Hospital
Bristol

Mandy Redgrove
Hospice Family and Group Worker
North Devon Hospice
Barnstaple

Audrey Smyth
Bereavement Group Worker
North Devon Hospice
Barnstaple

Francesca Thompson
Macmillan Nurse Consultant
Macmillan Cancer Relief

Mary Woods
Senior Clinical Nurse Specialist
   (Lymphoedema Services)
The Royal Marsden Hospital
Sutton

Acknowledgements

I would like to thank all of the authors for their enthusiasm, dedication, commitment and willingness to share their knowledge. Any success will be totally due to their inspiration and efforts. Special thanks must also go to Susanna Hill for giving up her time to read and comment on some chapters. To Jenny Penson, Louise (Lulu) Whitehead and David for their valuable comments and expertise. To Jon Hibberd for his evaluation and to Heidi Allen for having 'faith' in me – thank you. With many thanks to my medical and nursing colleagues who are always a source of inspiration and support. It is important to stress that any omissions and/or errors remain the sole responsibility of this editor.

Jo Cooper

To David for unending patience, support and understanding, and for continuously reminding me that 'all will be well'. Thank you.

To Philip, Marc and Caroline for making everything worthwhile.

To Joyce and Charlie, with all my love always.

PART ONE
Practical approaches to individual care

CHAPTER 1

Introduction to pain control

Trevor Mitten

Pre-reading exercise

1 What questions could you ask individuals about their pain? Write down your thoughts. Examples of the type of question useful in pain assessment are listed at the end of the chapter.
2 Think of a time when you, or someone close to you, were experiencing pain. What steps did you take to identify the cause of the pain and to control it?

At the end of the chapter, review your answers to see whether you explored all of the possible approaches, or if you could have achieved more effective pain control.

Assessing pain

In attempting to discuss pain control, the single most important thing is to ask the right questions and to listen to the answers. It is a primary function of pain assessment to ensure that the patient, relative(s) and health professional have an understanding both of what is being said and of what is not being said. Therefore, the first prerequisite for good pain control is a full and comprehensive history. One sentence from a patient can make a clear connection between how the individual is feeling and the type of pain that is being experienced. Once this is taken into account, pain control becomes more effective, and pain is easier to treat. Close observation of the individual's body language, and of expressions relating to disruption of the patient's normal activity, may reveal as much about the presence and nature of pain, as the presence and description of the pain itself. Examples of this may include the following:

- complaints of waking at night with discomfort;
- the patient sitting in a 'special chair' (it is common for people in pain to seek a chair that is perceived to reduce pain levels);
- propping with cushions or 'leaning' into the pain;
- use of the hand or other object(s) to apply pressure at the pain site;
- rubbing constantly at the pain site.

An essential aid to pain assessment is the patient's relative(s). It is imperative that their views are taken into account. There is a risk that the patient may not wish to be seen as complaining or weak, and thus pain may be under-reported. Indeed, it is not uncommon for pain to be 'eased' or to disappear altogether during conversation with the community professional. It is estimated that up to 25% of cancer sufferers have four or more pains.[1] The individual may experience pain in one area that originates from somewhere else; this is called referred pain.[2] It is important to ask if the individual is experiencing different types of pain, as they may well have more than one! Equally, it should be born in mind that the pain experienced might not be directly related to the cancer, although it is important to address *all* pain.

Regular reassessment and evaluation of pain is important. It should be regarded as a continuum and not a 'one-off' exercise. It may be that as one pain is controlled or eased, the individual becomes aware of another. Pain may also reappear later and or become transformed into a different type of pain altogether. The use of pain diaries or pain assessment tools is an important part of individual assessment and gives the patient a sense of control. Rating mechanisms such as a simple visual analogue scale may suffice, or the London Hospitals pain chart,[3] in which the individual draws the pain site on a 'body outline,' may be used.

The primary aims of pain control are:

- a good night's sleep;
- pain relief at rest;
- pain relief on movement, although this may be more difficult to achieve.

Patient's awareness of pain

How the patient expresses pain is important. They may say that there is no pain. This may be because they have adapted to chronic pain and cannot or do not yet acknowledge its presence. However, if the patient is asked whether there is any discomfort or aching, then pain may be acknowledged. It is common for patients to describe pain in terms of discomfort rather than directly to describe it as pain. This issue should be explored carefully with the patient and relatives, and must not be ignored.

Although it is accepted that the most reliable indicator of pain is related by the patient, it has been demonstrated that nurses tend not to rely on self-reporting.[4] If effective intervention in pain control is to be achieved, such practice must be reversed.

Rapidly increasing pain

At some stage, a rapid increase in the level of pain may be experienced. This often occurs during the final stages of life, and is very frightening for both the patient and their family, often causing feelings of anxiety and panic. Prompt review of the situation, a calm manner and appropriate intervention may help to allay some of the fears and concerns. The importance of awareness that such situations can arise and that they require prompt, effective management cannot be over-emphasised.

Analgesia may need to be increased rapidly, especially as the situation can change within the hour. Some practitioners express concern about how quickly the need for pain relief increases. The need for analgesia during terminal illness is often considerably greater than the level of analgesia used by the community professional on a routine basis within the community setting, which can be a source of anxiety for the professional. However, this is not a good reason for withholding adequate analgesia. Discussion within the multidisciplinary team will help to support the community professional.

Simple measures

Often nurses and doctors find that the focus is on medication, which is perceived as a panacea for the control of pain. However, simple measures can often be effective in pain control, such as the following:

- the use of a hot water bottle;
- a hot bath;
- a wheat bag or heat pad.

Such measures are simple and non-invasive. They are readily available and, most importantly, they empower the individual or carer to feel that they can do something to lessen the effects of pain themselves. The role of careful positioning and judicious use of pillows should not be underestimated. Other therapies will be discussed later in the chapter.

Compliance with treatment

For pain relief to be effective, it is essential that adequate time is spent explaining the need for strong opioid therapy. Allowing time for discussion is essential in order to allay fears and maximise compliance with medication. One reason for deferred prescribing of morphine is the concern that 'tolerance' may develop. However, evidence exists that the need for an increased dosage of opioids is associated with disease progression rather than pharmacological tolerance.[5]

Some individuals fear morphine dependency. However, in many cases the patient who is receiving high-dose opioids has effectively reduced or ceased medication, following treatment (e.g. radiotherapy or nerve blocks) with little or no effect.

Analgesic ladder

The World Health Organisation (WHO) analgesic ladder[6] is a useful guide to prescription of the appropriate level of analgesia (*see* Figure 1.1). This progresses from Step One, when the use of non-opioids such as paracetamol and non-steroidal anti-inflammatory drugs (e.g. ibuprofen) may be appropriate. If the pain remains uncontrolled although the maximum dose has been achieved, then progression to Step Two follows. A weak opioid such as co-proxamol or dihydrocodeine, with non-steroidal anti-inflammatory drug(s) and other adjuvants as appropriate, may be effective. After the maximum dose of Step Two drugs has been reached, then progression to Step Three is recommended. Step Three drugs include the strong opioids, such as morphine, prescribed with or without adjuvant drugs. (Note that adjuvant drugs are used to compliment other drugs and to maximise pain control, and they can be used at any step of the analgesic ladder.) It is important to stress that the WHO analgesic ladder is merely a guide to pain control. It is neither essential nor necessary to follow the ladder in all cases. In some instances, it may be more appropriate to prescribe Step Three drugs immediately – hence the need for a thorough assessment of pain.

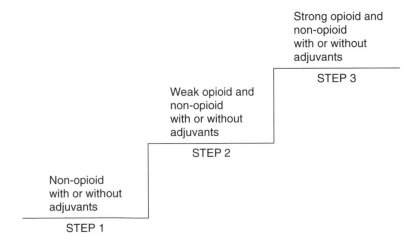

Figure 1.1 WHO three-step analgesic ladder.[6]

The use of opioids in pain control

Oral morphine is the strong opioid of choice for cancer pain.[1] Some patients, particularly the elderly, view it with suspicion. However, a clear and concise explanation of its uses and advantages over other medication is usually effective in obtaining compliance.[7] A regular laxative should always be prescribed prophylactically whenever morphine is used, as constipation is inevitable. Initially, an anti-emetic may be needed if nausea or vomiting is a problem.

Sedation can be problematic. However, the individual patient will adapt to the increased dose, and sedation decreases after 3 or 4 days. Morphine is best prescribed as regular dose medication. If prescribed only 'as required', it has been found to be less effective.[8] This requires careful explanation to both the patient and their relative(s). Oral morphine is available as:

● solution (Oramorph) – quick release;
● tablet (Sevredol) – quick release;
● tablet (morphine sulphate tablet, MST) – sustained release, administered 12-hourly;
● MST suspension – powder, administered 12-hourly.

There are several preparations of liquid morphine available. The most common of these is Oramorph solution, which is quickly absorbed and is useful for breakthrough pain. In addition, it can be used to assess opioid need before switching to a long-acting morphine. The standard strengths of Oramorph solution are 10 mg/5 mL and 100 mg/5 mL. To reduce the sharp taste, it can be mixed with a sweet cordial.

Single-dose twist-top plastic vial preparations of Oramorph (unit dose vials) are available, which are useful in cases where manual dexterity is a problem. The drug is prepared in three strengths of 10 mg/5 mL, 30 mg/5 mL and 100 mg/5 mL. It can be administered as a fluid directly into the mouth. In addition, there is a tablet form of quick-release morphine (Sevredol, with tablets available in strengths of 10 mg, 20 mg and 50 mg).

It is generally recommended that treatment with morphine is commenced using a quick-acting preparation before converting to a sustained-release preparation.[9] This enables rapid titration to the therapeutic level.

Oral doses for breakthrough pain can be offered every 60–90 minutes as appropriate.[10] The rescue dose for breakthrough pain is one-third of the 12-hourly dose of sustained-release morphine. It is important to review the effect of the morphine and the pain regularly. The dose should be increased as appropriate, taking into account all of the rescue doses taken within a 24-hour period. If additional doses are required several times during the day, this suggests that the regular dose needs to be increased.[1]

Morphine sulphate tablets (MST) in a sustained-release formulation are available in

Table 1.1 Example of night-time morphine doses for breakthrough pain

Morphine	Night-time dose for breakthrough pain
Up to 30 mg	Double the dose
Over 30 mg	Increase the dose by 50%

strengths of 5 mg, 10 mg, 15 mg, 30 mg, 60 mg, 100 mg and 200 mg, and are suitable for twice-daily administration.

If the patient was receiving a weak opioid, then commence with 10 mg, 4-hourly or 30 mg sustained-release preparation 12-hourly.[1] These doses may need to be reduced in the elderly frail adult.[1]

Pain is frequently problematic at night, often waking the patient. One method of avoiding this is to give an increased dose of Oramorph at bedtime (Table 1.1 gives an example of doses).

When considering increasing the dose of morphine, it is recommended[1] that the dose is increased after 24 hours if the pain is not relieved by 90% (e.g. from 5 to 10 mg, from 10 to 15 mg, from 20 to 30 mg). In addition, there is a strong case for using adjuvant drugs when administering strong opioids. Different types of pain, such as bone or nerve pain, respond to different types of medication.

Common side-effects of morphine use

Common side-effects of morphine include constipation, nausea and vomiting, drowsiness, and bad dreams and hallucinations (Table 1.2).

Table 1.2 Common side-effects of morphine and their treatment

Morphine side effect	Treatment
Constipation	Laxatives (e.g. codanthramer, senna, lactulose); titrate as necessary
Nausea/vomiting	Anti-emetics (e.g. haloperidol 500 microgrammes–1.5 mg three times daily). Metoclopramide (10 mg three times daily). Nausea often settles after a few days. Review frequently
Drowsiness	No treatment. Effect wears off after a few days but may recur temporarily after a dose increase. Clear explanation to patient and their relative(s) is essential. If pain is controlled, the dose can be reduced
Bad dreams/hallucinations	Not so common. Assess opioid toxicity and reduce dose if appropriate. Haloperidol (1.5 mg three times daily) can be prescribed, or alternatively switch to a different strong opioid

Long-acting strong opioids

There are several long-acting morphine preparations available on the market, together with other strong opioids, which are summarised in Table 1.3.

Table 1.3   Other long-acting opioid preparations

Drug	Starting dose	Indications for use
MST suspension	10–30 mg twice a day for opioid-naïve patients or those previously on weak opioids	MST suspension is a sachet of powder which when mixed with water, forms a suspension that the patient drinks. This is useful if swallowing tablets is a problem. It can also be syringed down a gastrostomy tube. It is available in a variety of doses up to 200-mg sachets, but is difficult to mix without forming lumps. To ensure even distribution of the mix, use 10–20 mL of very hot water as the base, and sprinkle the powder on slowly while stirring gently. Ensure that the mix is cool before administration
Morcap	20 mg once daily (also licensed for 12-hourly administration)	This is a capsule form of morphine that can be opened and sprinkled onto food
MXL	30 mg once daily	This is a once daily capsule preparation of sustained-release morphine
Hydromorphone	4 mg 12-hourly	Can be opened and sprinkled onto soft, cold food. This is often used in rotation of opioids
Methadone	Specialist advice is needed pre-prescription	Used in opioid rotation for severe pain. It has a long half-life in the body (i.e. it takes a long time to be broken down), and can accumulate to toxic levels. May be beneficial for neuropathic pain. As an opioid rotation agent it has a greater higher delta-receptor effect than morphine, and a wide spectrum of activity
Fentanyl TTS, transdermal fentanyl patch	25 microgramme every 3 days for opioid-naïve patients	Stable severe pain (*see* pp. 10–12 for further discussion)
Oxycodone	30 mg suppository 8-hourly	Useful for patients who are unable to tolerate oral medication. This is given as a suppository, providing 6–8 hours of relief

Prescribing consideration

Consideration must be given to possible side-effects related to opioid use. These may include the following:

- possible toxic effects;
- intolerable side-effects (e.g. constipation, nausea, vomiting, sedation), which may outweigh the benefits;
- renal failure – accumulation of morphine metabolites;
- decreasing effectiveness of a strong opioid; switching to an alternative strong opioid may reduce this effect – this is referred to as 'rotation of opioids';[11]
- compliance – fear of the drug and an unwillingness to take morphine. Alternative opioids may elicit compliance.

Diamorphine profile

Chemically, diamorphine consists of two morphine molecules locked together. It is available in the UK and is used in preference to morphine for subcutaneous infusions. It has a much higher solubility in solutions. As a strong opioid, it is the preferred choice for use in a syringe driver for subcutaneous infusion. Diamorphine is twice as potent as morphine when administered by injection.[1]

Converting from morphine to diamorphine

When converting from morphine to diamorphine, the following factors will need to be considered.[1]

- When converting from oral morphine to subcutaneous morphine, halve the oral dose.
- When converting from oral morphine to subcutaneous diamorphine, give one-third of the oral dose.
- When converting from oral diamorphine to subcutaneous diamorphine, halve the oral dose.

Increments in dose should be in the range 25–50%. Additional subcutaneous doses for breakthrough pain should be 50–100% of the equivalent 4-hourly dose.[12]

Fentanyl

Fentanyl is available as a patch (durogesic) or as an injection that can be given intravenously or by syringe driver for morphine-intolerant individuals. The transdermal patch is widely used and will thus be the focus of this chapter. The fentanyl patch is clear in appearance and is applied to the skin. Patches are changed every 72 hours.

Fentanyl patches have been shown to reduce the risk of constipation and also have value in reducing the daytime somnolence caused by morphine.[13]

Fentanyl is of clinical value at the end of life when a non-oral route is preferred. If a fentanyl patch is already *in situ*, then it is unnecessary to switch to another strong opioid unless pain is escalating rapidly or a syringe driver is required to control other troublesome symptoms.

It is essential that patients with fentanyl patches are prescribed quick-release morphine for breakthrough pain. This must be given in the correct dose for the patch size, and the dose should be increased whenever the patch size is increased. This process needs to be explained to the patient and their family so that they understand the rationale. Fentanyl can take from 12 to 24 hours to achieve maximum blood concentration.[12] The patches are available in four strengths:

- 25 microgramme/hour;
- 50 microgramme/hour;
- 75 microgramme/hour;
- 100 microgramme/hour.

If the patient is currently receiving morphine sulphate tablets (MST), the fentanyl patch is applied with the last oral dose of MST.[12]

Areas requiring consideration

Some reports have indicated that the fentanyl patch only lasts for 2 days (the normal application period is 3 days).[14] If pain control is maximised at 2 days but decreases on day 3, the patch can be changed on the second day.

Counselling is essential for the patient and their relative(s) throughout this procedure. Verbal and written guidance about the application of the patch is essential. Careful explanation of the potential side-effects will ease anxiety and aid compliance. Patients do find the patches advantageous, as the need for oral medication is reduced, comfort is increased, and the daily reminder relating to health may be decreased.

Dosages

The normal starting dose is a 25 microgramme patch. If an individual is converting from 4-hourly oral morphine to fentanyl, the morphine should be continued for 12 hours[15] while the blood concentration achieves maximum saturation.

Recommendations for converting from oral morphine to a fentanyl patch (Table 1.4), have been made by Back.[12] For breakthrough pain it is recommended[12,16] that the fentanyl patch is divided by 5 (Patch/5) to give the dose in milligrams of diamorphine administered subcutaneously.

Twycross and colleagues[15] suggest that, when converting fentanyl patches to continuous subcutaneous diamorphine given via a syringe driver, the following apply.

- Give half the patch strength as milligrams per 24 hours rounded up to a convenient ampoule size.
- After 24 hours, give the whole of the previous patch strength as milligrams per 24 hours rounded up to a convenient ampoule size.

Table 1.4 Back's fentanyl recommendation for conversion[12]

Oral morphine/24 hours	Fentanyl patch/hour
Naïve	25 microgramme
<135 mg	25 microgramme
135–225 mg	50 microgramme
225–315 mg	75 microgramme
315–405 mg	100 microgramme
405–495 mg	125 microgramme
495–585 mg	150 microgramme
585–675 mg	175 microgramme
675–765 mg	200 microgramme
765–855 mg	225 microgramme
855–945 mg	250 microgramme
945–1035 mg	275 microgramme
1035–1125 mg	300 microgramme

Side-effects

A small number of patients who switch from morphine to fentanyl patches experience a state of clamminess, sweating, nausea and restlessness[16] within 24-hours of switching over. This can be due to morphine withdrawal. One or two doses of quick-release morphine will alleviate these symptoms while adjustment to the new medication takes place.

New developments

The use of a fentanyl lozenge on a stick may be one of the future developments in pain control. At the time of writing, the outcome of clinical trials is still awaited. The lozenge is impregnated with a specific strength of fentanyl. This is sucked and the drug is absorbed via the mucous membrane in the mouth. In American trials it has been suggested that 'transmucosal fentanyl' offers greater control of breakthrough pain with an increased analgesic effect.[17] One study found significant effects after 5 minutes.[18]

Opioid rotation

Inadequate pain control with escalating opioid doses in the presence of dose-limiting toxic effects, including hallucinations, confusion, hyperalgesia, myoclonus, sedation and nausea, may be a problem in some cases. When the patient requires increasing doses of a strong analgesic, benefit may be obtained from drug rotation. Adjuvant drugs should always be considered when prescribing morphine (or indeed any other strong opioid), as this may reduce the need for escalating doses of these drugs.

Outcome surveys[19] have demonstrated that the toxic effects of opioids can be relieved by opioid rotation. This can be achieved by substituting a different opioid in an equi-analgesic dose. One area of concern has been the conversion to methadone. The latter drug has been demonstrated to be more potent than was previously suggested. Specialist advice should be sought if rotating to this opioid.

Opioid-unresponsive pain

Some pains are not fully responsive to opioids. These include:

- bone pain;
- nerve (neurogenic) pain.

Careful listening to the patient's or relative's description of the pain can provide vital information relating to the type of pain.

Bone pain

This may consist of aching joints, sometimes described as 'toothache'. Heaviness may be experienced in the back or hips, which is often worse on movement. Bone pain may arise for a variety of reasons, including osteoarthritis or pathological fracture, and it may be due to bone metastases.

Cancers that are likely to cause bone metastases include the following:

- breast;
- prostate;
- multiple myeloma;
- bronchus;
- kidney.

The first-line drugs of choice are non-steroidal anti-inflammatory drugs (NSAIDs). NSAIDs inhibit prostaglandin synthesis by inhibiting the enzyme cyclo-oxygenase.[16]

Table 1.5 provides some guidance on the use of anti-inflammatory drugs.

NSAIDs have been reported to help to control bone pain in 80% of patients.[20] It is worth rotating to different non-steroidal drugs if one particular drug does not work.[21] Ketorolac is a relatively new NSAID which is available in tablet form or can be administered by intravenous or subcutaneous injection.[22,23] Administration via a syringe driver is beneficial if other oral NSAIDS have failed.[24] This can be attributed to ketorolac's dual anti-inflammatory and analgesic effect.[25] The improved absorption via the parenteral route will also play a role.

Table 1.5   Anti-inflammatory drugs and suggested doses

Anti-inflammatory drug	Dosage
Aspirin	600 mg four times daily
Ibuprofen	200–600 mg four times daily, or Brufen Retard two tablets daily (800 mg)
Flurbiprofen (Froben)	50–100 mg three times daily; also available as suppositories (100 mg)
Diclofenac (Voltarol)	Oral formulation 150 mg/day; also available as suppositories 50 mg/100 mg
Ketorolac (Toradol)	30 mg/day by oral route; 60–120 mg/day by syringe driver
Diclofenac with misoprostol (Arthrotec)	One tablet (50 mg/200 microgramme) three times daily, or one tablet (75 mg/200 μg) twice daily

NSAIDS tend to cause gastric irritation. Adjuvant treatment with misoprostol 200 microgramme daily, or omeprazole 20 mg once daily, should be considered.[26]

The use of biphosphonates such as pamidronate in cases of bone pain is encouraging.[27] Even when individuals have a normal calcium level,[28] treatment with a biphosphonate such as pamidronate (60–90 mg IV[29] every 4–6 weeks) can markedly reduce the pain from bone metastases. Higher doses can be given less often, with a report of 120 mg of Pamidronate lasting for 3–6 months.[30]

The use of injections of strontium[89 TM] for the relief of metastatic bone pain is becoming widespread, and is indicated for patients with prostate or breast cancer. Strontium follows the pathway of calcium, delivering local radiotherapy to metastatic sites. Bone metastases concentrate and preserve more strontium[89 TM] than normal tissues.

Nerve pain

This is described as stabbing, shooting, burning pain or pins and needles. The pain often follows nerve pathways such as that of the facial nerve (e.g. trigeminal neuralgia) or thoracic nerve (e.g. shingles). It is not fully controlled by opioids,[31] and often responds well to antidepressant medication (e.g. amitriptyline or dothiepin — particularly if the sensation is 'burning'). If these drugs are not effective, the second stage often involves adding an anticonvulsant drug such as carbamazepine or sodium valproate (Epilim),[32] (particularly if the sensation is 'stabbing'). If neither of these work, Gabapentin has proved useful. If the nerve pain is resistant to all of these measures, the use of anti-arrhythmic drugs such as flecainide may be considered.[33] Discussion with the multidisciplinary team and specialist palliative care teams is important in order to achieve a common approach and optimise outcome.

amitryptline - nerve

Other treatments for nerve pain include the following:

- epidural injection;[34]
- coeliac plexus block;
- chemical nerve destruction with phenol;
- surgical nerve destruction (e.g. cordotomy).

The flow chart on opioid-unresponsive pain shown in Figure 1.2 indicates considerations and actions for addressing these types of pain.

Steroids in pain control

The use of steroids in pain control needs to be weighed against the side-effects. Steroids can be effective in pain control if used appropriately. Dexamethasone is often the steroid of choice.[16] The use of steroids in the control of pain is indicated in the following:

- raised intra-cranial pressure;
- spinal cord compression;
- bone pain.[16]

Prescribing and administering steroids

The steroid dexamethasone is frequently prescribed in palliative care. It crosses the blood–brain barrier, so is useful in patients with cerebral tumours. It is approximately seven times more potent than prednisolone, so fewer tablets are needed.[16] Dexamethasone tablets can be crushed and made into a suspension with warm water, rendering them easier to swallow. Steroids may cause nocturnal insomnia, and once or twice daily (morning and lunchtime) administration is preferable[35] to an evening or nocte dose. To help prevent dyspepsia or ulcers, an H_2-antagonist can be added which helps to protect the gut.

The side-effects of steroid use include the following:

- gastric irritation or ulceration;
- water retention;
- immunosuppression;
- steroid psychosis;
- oral candidiasis;
- insomnia;
- thinning of the skin;
- hypertension;
- steroid-induced diabetes.

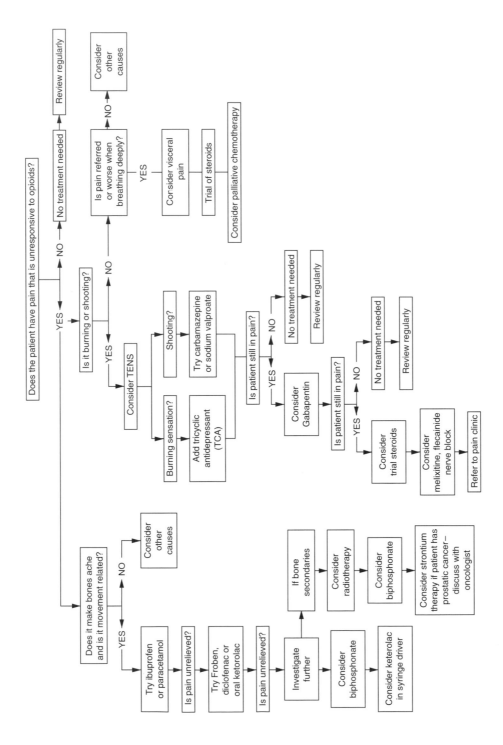

Figure 1.2 Flow chart for opioid-unresponsive pain.

Visceral pain

Visceral pain can be worse on taking a deep breath. It can present as an excruciating pain when an organ cannot swell to accommodate a tumour due to the presence of inflexible viscera containing the organ. The most common example is liver pain due to metastases in the liver causing liver capsule stretch. Treatment is usually with morphine and high-dose steroids (dexamethasone 8–16 mg/day), which reduces peri-tumour oedema. Palliative radiotherapy or chemotherapy may also be indicated.

Non-pharmacological control of pain

The use of trans-cutaneous electrical nerve stimulation (TENS) machines has been found to be beneficial in both hospital and community settings. It has been reported that in 47% of patients after the use of a TENS machine a 50% reduction in pain intensity had been achieved.[36] Careful instruction and regular monitoring are necessary.

The following types of pain are often helped by TENS:

- back pain;
- rib metastases or fractures;
- sciatica;
- post-herpetic neuralgia;
- phantom limb pain;
- musculo-skeletal pain;
- diabetic neuropathy.

TENS should be applied by an appropriately trained practitioner. Initially a period of 20–30 minutes should be used to test the effectiveness of the treatment. This can then be increased according to the response. It is inadvisable to use the machine all the time, but a period of up to 12 hours a day may be required if the patient is not receiving any other analgesia.[37]

TENS works by blocking the transmission of painful stimuli (referred to as the 'gate theory') by increasing activity in the large 'A' fibres and decreasing activity in the smaller pain fibres. It is suggested that this releases endorphins in the dorsal horn. The settings vary according to the patient's pain. A starting frequency of 4–80 Hz, and pulse duration of 200 microseconds is a good baseline.

It is recommended that TENS electrodes are not placed across the heart or the side of the neck near the carotid arteries, or on areas of broken or irradiated skin, as this could affect the heart rate or cause electrode burns. It is important to check the pads regularly to ensure that there is sufficient electrode gel. The electrodes and electrode leads should also be replaced periodically as they do wear out.

It is important to read the manufacturer's instructions carefully before commencing TENS treatment.

Psychological approaches

Pain can be described in terms of physical, spiritual, emotional and psychological factors, and has been referred to as 'total pain'.[38] The patient will need ongoing assessment and counselling with regard to issues such as family problems and religious or spiritual needs, in addition to analgesia. It is acknowledged that a state of anxiety increases the intensity of pain.[39] Diazepam can aid relaxation. It has been recorded that lorazepam (0.5–1 mg 6-hourly as needed) can also be helpful. Given sublingually, it has been reported to be effective.[40] It is important to be aware that psychological pain is real pain, and it should not be overlooked or dismissed.

'Coping strategies' such as distraction therapy, visualisation and imagery[41] empower the individual and enable better coping skills to be developed.

Relaxation and visualisation

Individuals who are in pain or who feel fear may become tense and agitated. For such patients, relaxation may be helpful. One definition of relaxation is 'a state of relative freedom from both anxiety and skeletal muscle tension'.[41] Relaxation can be effective in conjunction with other interventions (e.g. drug therapy) in reducing tension. Simple breathing exercises can be taught during counselling.

Visualisation involves taking control of one's thoughts and distancing oneself from unpleasant situations.

These techniques can benefit the patient by aiding sleep, promoting management of stress and pain, and reducing anxiety and depression.[42] It may be appropriate to involve the community psychiatric nurse during assessment and for specialist guidance.

Other therapeutic interventions

These may include the following:

- physiotherapy;
- aromatherapy;
- hypnotherapy;
- osteopathy;
- acupuncture;
- massage.

Conclusions

The key to effective pain control is continuous assessment. Effective intervention involves taking action immediately when pain is identified. Being aware of new interventions and developments in drug therapy is a prerequisite of good practice.

The relative(s) should never be excluded from the process of pain assessment. It is extremely distressing to see one's partner, sibling or child in chronic unrelieved pain. Inclusion, support, guidance and the opportunity to discuss how the individual feels are imperative if therapeutic intervention is to be successful.

Regular review is the best policy. Involving the multidisciplinary team throughout therapeutic interventions will ensure a team approach to the identified problems and will improve intervention, understanding of the nature of the pain and communication. It is important to continue supporting the individual even when interventions have not proved successful, as merely being present is a therapeutic intervention in itself.

When assessing and planning intervention related to pain and its control, *listening* and *correct interpretation* are the primary tools which are most effective for all community professionals.

Chapter 1:   Questions

1 A patient says that their pain is burning and continuous in nature. What type of pain do you think this might indicate?
2 What drug treatment might be prescribed for nerve pain?
3 What are the 'Three Steps' in the WHO analgesic ladder?
4 List three non-pharmacological treatments that may help to relieve pain.
5 Identify three non-verbal indicators that the patient may be in pain.
6 What are the common side-effects of morphine?
7 When may fentanyl patches be indicated?
8 When should we not listen to the patient and their relative(s)?

References

1   Twycross R (1999) *Introducing Palliative Care* (3e). Radcliffe Medical Press, Oxford.

2   Cambell J (1995) Making sense of . . . pain management. *Nursing Times.* **91**: 34–5.

3   Collins S and Parker E (1983) *An Introduction to Nursing.* Macmillan Publishing. London.

4   Jacox AJ (1979) Assessing pain. *Am J Nursing.* **79**: 895–900.

5   Collin E, Poulain P, Gauvain-Piquard A *et al.* (1993) Is disease progression the major factor in morphine 'tolerance' in cancer pain treatment? *Pain.* **55**: 319–26.

6   World Health Organisation (1996) *Cancer Pain Relief* (2e). World Health Organisation, Geneva.

7   Carr E (1997) Myths and fears about pain-relieving drugs. *Nursing Times.* **93**: 50–1.

8   Hanks G, Hoskin P, Aherne G *et al.* (1987) Explanation for potency of repeated oral doses of morphine? *Lancet.* **1**: 723–5.

9   Hanks G, De Conno F, Ripamonti C *et al.* (1996). Morphine in cancer pain: modes of administration. *BMJ.* **312**: 823–6.

10   Hanks G and Doyle D (1994) *Oxford Textbook of Palliative Care* (2e). Oxford University Press, Oxford.

11   Stoutz N, Bruera E and Suarez-Almazor M (1995) Opioid rotation for toxicity reduction in terminal cancer individuals. *J Pain Symptom Management.* **10**: 378–84.

12   Back IN (1998) *Palliative Medicine Handbook.* I Back, Glamorgan.

13   Ahmedzai S and Brooks D (1997) Transdermal fentanyl versus sustained-release oral morphine in cancer pain: preference, efficacy, and quality of life. The TTS-Fentanyl Comparative Trial Group. *J Pain Symptom Management.* **13**: 254–61.

14   Payne R, Chandler S and Einhaus M (1995) Guidelines for the clinical use of trans-dermal Fentanyl. *Anticancer Drugs.* **6 (Suppl 3)**: 50–3.

15   Twycross R, Wilcock A and Thorp S (1998) *PCF1 Palliative Care Formulary.* Radcliffe Medical Press, Oxford.

16   Twycross R (1997) *Symptom Management in Advanced Cancer* (2e). Radcliffe Medical Press, Oxford.

17   Portenoy R, Payne R, Coluzzi P *et al.* (1999) Oral transmucosal fentanyl citrate (OFTC) for the treatment of breakthrough pain in cancer patients: a controlled dose titration study. *Pain.* **79**: 303–12.

18   Farrar JT, Cleary J, Rauck R *et al.* (1998) Oral transmucosal fentanyl citrate: rando-mized, double-blinded, placebo-controlled trial for treatment of breakthrough pain in cancer patients. *J Nat Cancer Inst.* **90**: 611–6.

19   http://www.meb.unibonn.de/cancernet/304470.html#9_PHARMACOLOGICMANAGE-MENT (Internet reference for opiate rotation accessed 03/01/2000).

20   Kaye P (1992) *A–Z of Hospice and Palliative Medicine.* EPL Publications, Northampton.

21   Roberts A (1997) Drugs used for pain relief in palliative care. *Prof Nurse.* **13**: 91–5.

22   Toscani F, Piva L, Corli O *et al.* (1994) Keterolac versus diclofenic sodium in cancer pain. *Arzeneim-forsch-drug-res.* **44**: 550–4.

23   Buckley M and Brogden R (1990) Keterolac: a review of its pharmacodynamic and pharmacokinetic properties and therapeutic potential. *Drugs.* **39**: 86–109.

24   Blackwell N, Bangham L, Hughes M *et al.* (1993) Subcutaneous keterolac – a new devel-opment in pain control. *Palliative Med.* **7**: 63–5.

25   Micaela M, Brogen B and Brogen R (1990) Keterolac – a review of its pharmacodynamic and pharmacokinetic properties and therapeutic potential. *Drugs.* **39**: 86–109.

26   Myers K (1999) What's new about NSAIDs? *Cont Med Educ Bull Palliative Med.* **1**: 31–3.

27   Williams J and Corcoran G (1996) *Palliative Care Prescribing* (Drug Information Leaflet No. 110). North-West Drug Information Service and Aintree Hospital NHS Trust, Liverpool.

28   Regnard C and Tempest S (1998) *A Guide to Symptom Relief in Advanced Disease* (4e). Hochland and Hochland, Manchester.

29   Ripamonti C, Fulfaro F, Ticozzi C *et al.* (1998) Role of pamidronate disodium in the treatment of metastatic bone disease. *Tumori*. **84**: 442–55.

30   Purohit OP, Anthony C, Radstone CR *et al.* (1994) High-dose intravenous pamidronate for metastatic bone pain. *Br J Cancer*. **70**: 554–8.

31   Gilbert J (1993) Opioid-resistant cancer pain. In: *RCGP Members' Reference Book*. RCGP, London.

32   Niffin P, McQuay H, Jadad A and Moore A (1995) Anticonvulsant drugs for management of pain: a systematic review. *BMJ*. **31**: 1047–52.

33   Sykes J, Johnson R and Hanks G (1997) Difficult pain problems. *BMJ*. **315**: 867.

34   Wood P, Rushby C and Ahmedzai S (1992) Epidural steroid injections for malignant pain. *J Cancer Care*. **1**, 139–44.

35   Edwards A and Gerrard G (1998) The management of cerebral metastases. *Eur J Palliative Care*. **5**: 7–11.

36   Johnson MI, Ashton CH and Thompson JW (1991) An in-depth study of long-term users of transcutaneous electrical nerve stimulation (TENS). Implications for the use of TENS. *Pain*. **44**: 221–9.

37   Mitchell A and Kafai S (1997) Patient education in TENS pain management. *Prof Nurse*. **12**: 804–7.

38   Saunders C (1990) *Hospice and Palliative Care – an Interdisciplinary Approach*. Edward Arnold, London.

39   Stimmel B (1997) *Pain and Its Relief Without Addiction*. The Haworth Medical Press, New York.

40   Kaye P (1995) *A–Z Pocketbook of Symptom Control*. EPL Publications, Northampton.

41   Waugh L (1988) Psychological aspects of cancer pain. *Prof Nurse*. **3**: 504–8.

42   McCaffrey M and Beebe A (1994) Pain. In: J Latham (ed) *Clinical Manual for Nursing Practice*. Mosby and Times Mirror International Publishing, London.

To learn more

McCaffrey M and Beebe A (1994) Pain. In: J Latham (ed) *Clinical Manual for Nursing Practice*. Mosby and Times Mirror International Publishing, London.

Regnard C and Tempest S (1998) *A Guide to Symptom Relief in Advanced Disease* (4e). Hochland and Hochland, Manchester.

Roxanne Pain Institute: www.pain.roxanne.com/main.html

Turk D and Melzack R (1992) *Handbook of Pain Assessment*. Guilford Press, New York.

Twycross R (1994) *Pain Relief in Advanced Cancer*. Churchill Livingstone, Edinburgh.

Twycross R, Wilcock A and Thorp S (1998) *PCF1 Palliative Care Formulary*. Radcliffe Medical Press, Oxford.

Williams M (1989) Some psychological aspects of pain. In: J Latham (ed) *Pain Control*. Austen Cornish, London.

Chapter 1:   Answers to pre-reading exercise

- Is the pain constant or does it come and go?
- What makes the pain worse?
- What makes the pain better?
- Is the pain worse on movement?
- Is the pain worse when lying down?
- Is the pain always in the same place or does it move around?
- Does the pain disturb your sleep?
- Does heat relieve your pain?
- What words do you use to describe your pain?

Chapter 1:   Answers

1 Nerve pain.
2 A tricyclic antidepressant and/or an anticonvulsant.
3 Step 1: non-opioid and adjuvants. Step 2: weak opioid, non-opioid and adjuvants. Step 3: strong opioid, non-opioid and adjuvants.
4 TENS machine, acupuncture, massage, aromatherapy, physiotherapy.
5 Holding the site of pain, rubbing the site of pain, leaning into the pain, applying pressure to the site of pain, sitting on a 'special chair,' waking at night with discomfort, propping with a cushion.
6 Constipation, nausea and vomiting, drowsiness.
7 If a non-oral route is indicated, if the patient has intractable constipation, or to gain compliance.
8 Never!

CHAPTER 2

Symptom control

Susanna Hill

Introduction

The management of symptoms presented by patients with life-threatening disease is pivotal to the role of the specialist health worker in palliative medicine. The approach should be holistic, examining the physical, social, psychological and spiritual dimensions of any problem, and it should involve both the patient and the carer.[1]

General principles of symptom control

Patients with life-threatening illness can present with many different symptoms. Box 2.1 lists those most frequently encountered, together with their prevalence in a hospice population.

Box 2.1: Prevalence of symptoms most frequently encountered in patients with life-threatening illness

Pain	82%
Nausea and vomiting	59%
Dyspnoea	51%
Constipation	51%
Weakness	64%
Anorexia	64%
Depression	40%
Confusion	20%

Frequency of symptoms in patients with advanced cancer.[2]

The patient who presents with multiple symptoms can be a daunting prospect for the palliative care professional – where does one start? A systematic approach can help to identify priorities, and enable a diagnosis to be made and appropriate treatment initiated.

The following sequence of steps should enable you to determine a reasonable management strategy for any symptom presented. Case studies involving different symptoms then demonstrate how to use this system. Throughout each section different learning points will be highlighted, and at the end of each section there will be several selected questions designed to help the reader to review the important points in the preceding section.

The sequence of steps to be used is as follows.

1 List the symptoms to be dealt with.
2 Prioritise (i.e. set the patient's agenda) – the patient, not the doctor or nurse, decides which symptom to deal with first.
3 List the possible causes of the symptom.
   Is it due to the illness, the treatment or other causes?
4 Establish the probable diagnosis.
   Take a *full* history, examine the patient properly and carry out any relevant investigations.
   Pay attention to detail, particularly in the history.
5 Establish the patient's understanding of the problem.
6 Discuss with the patient what you feel is the most likely cause of the problem, and use plain English, not medical jargon.
   'Align' yourself with the patient[3] by providing them with enough information in an understandable form for you to be able to discuss the problems on an equal basis.
7 Decide on an appropriate treatment.
   Think medical intervention vs. non-medical intervention (e.g. morphine vs. TENS or acupuncture, or all three!).
8 Individualise the treatment to the patient.
9 Set realistic goals for treatment – maintain hope.[4]
10 Assess the response of the patient to treatment.
11 Review! Review! Review!
   The patient's situation is always changing. Are the symptoms the same? Is the treatment working?

Box 2.2:   Self-assessment questions

- Categorise the causes of symptoms into three general groups.
- List the 11 steps used in determining the management of symptoms.

'I feel really sick' – nausea and vomiting

Case 2.1

Mrs Brown, an anxious 55-year-old lady, was diagnosed as having carcinoma of the pancreas 9 months ago. Recently she started vomiting copious amounts. She is also complaining of a swollen abdomen and back pain. Her current medication is morphine sulphate slow-release tablets (MST), 120 mg twice daily (bd), and metoclopramide, 10 mg four times a day as necessary (qds prn).

Step 1 – list of problem symptoms

Nausea, vomiting, pain and distended abdomen.

Step 2 – prioritise the symptoms

Nausea.
For many patients this is more unpleasant than recurrent vomiting.

Step 3 – list the possible causes

Box 2.3:	Possible causes of symptoms in Case 2.1	
Illness	● Gastrointestinal tract	– Cancer of the oesophagus
		– Cancer of the stomach
		– Squashed stomach syndrome
		– Cancer of the pancreas
		– Outlet obstruction
		– Constipation
		– Bowel obstruction
	● Cerebral	– Taste/smell
		– Fear/anxiety
		– Cerebral secondaries
		– Vestibular
	● Metabolic	– Hypercalcaemia

		– Uraemia
		– Tumour toxins
Treatment		– Chemotherapy
		– Radiotherapy
	• Other drugs	– Cerebral effect (e.g. opioids, antibiotics)
		– Gastric effect (e.g. steroids, NSAIDs)
Other causes		– Peptic ulcer
		– Gall-bladder disease
		– Reflux oesophagitis
		– Renal disease
		– Labyrinthitis

Step 4 – establish the probable diagnosis

Box 2.4:   Establishing the probable diagnosis

History

- Is there any obvious relationship (e.g. with food or pain) – peptic ulcer?
- Is it projectile or faeculent – high obstruction?
- Did it start with certain medication (e.g. morphine, digoxin, NSAIDs)?
- Do certain situations or events trigger it (e.g. hospital, chemotherapy)?

Examination

- Look for masses, hepatomegaly, jaundice, ascites, constipation, etc.

Investigations

- These include a full blood count, urea and electrolyte levels, calcium, glucose level, liver function tests, abdominal X-ray and gastroscopy.

Mrs Brown's vomiting did not have any obvious diagnostic features. It occurred at any time of day, was profuse but not obviously projectile, and was accompanied by almost constant nausea. She had a distended abdomen with shifting dullness, was slightly jaundiced, and had a hard, irregular, palpable liver edge. She was clinically diagnosed as having ascites and hepatic metastases. Her basic blood indices and biochemistry were measured. These confirmed a mild anaemia, with haemoglobin (Hb) of 9.5 g/dL, and slightly raised bilirubin and alkaline phosphatase levels, consistent with a mild obstructive jaundice.

The possible causes of Mrs Brown's nausea and vomiting were thought to be as follows:

- ascites;
- hepatomegaly;
- squashed stomach syndrome;
- hepatic disease;
- tumour toxins;
- drugs (opioid);
- anxiety.

Steps 5 and 6 – establish the patient's understanding of the problem and discuss possible causes

Mrs Brown did not have any ideas about why her nausea was so bad, but she did express anxiety that it must mean progression of her tumour. She had little belief that she would ever feel any better.

Step 7 – decide on the most relevant treatment

To determine the most appropriate treatment, an understanding of the neurotransmitters and pathways involved in nausea and vomiting is necessary. The vomiting reflex is initiated from the integrated vomiting centre (VC) in the hindbrain. This sends impulses via the efferent fibres of the vagal nerve to the stomach and upper gastrointestinal tract to cause vomiting. Afferent pathways carry signals from different areas of the body to the vomiting centre. Each pathway acts centrally via a different neurotransmitter. Drugs that block the neurotransmitter receptors inhibit the passage of the afferent signal to the vomiting centre.

Box 2.5:   Key point

Knowledge of the peripheral pathways and central neurotransmitters which trigger nausea and vomiting will enable you to choose the most effective anti-emetic.

Treatment options

Look for any causes that can be specifically treated, such as:

- constipation;
- gastritis;
- raised intracranial pressure;
- oropharyngeal candida;
- hypercalcaemia;
- drugs.

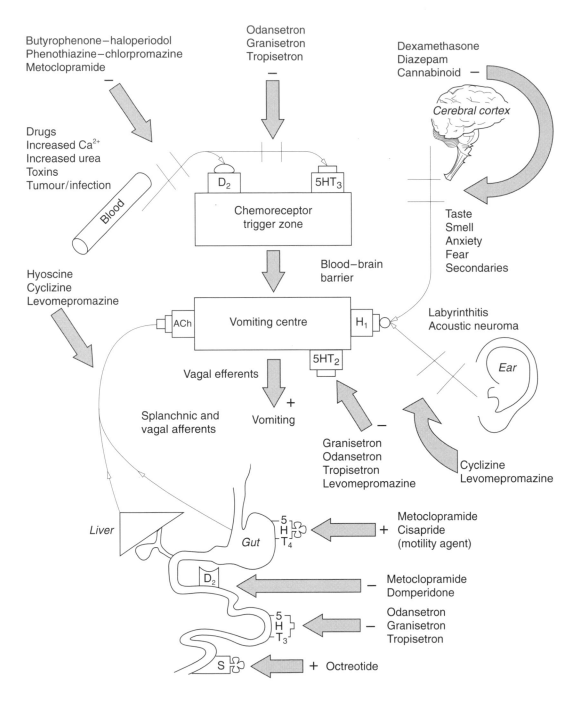

Figure 2.1 Triggers, pathways and neurotransmitter inhibitors involved in nausea and vomiting. Receptors: D_2, dopamine; S, somatostatin; ACh, muscarinic cholinergic.

If the patient is still symptomatic, choose an appropriate anti-emetic based on the most likely cause of nausea and vomiting (*see* Figure 2.1). The anti-emetic chosen should block the receptor which responds to the neurotransmitter for that pathway. If the first drug used is unsuccessful, choose an anti-emetic from another group.[5] If it is partially successful, consider adding the second drug.

A stepwise approach to the management of nausea and vomiting can be adopted that is similar to the analgesic ladder used in pain control.[6]

1 **Metoclopramide** acts peripherally as a motility agent and centrally as an anti-dopaminergic agent, acting at the chemoreceptor trigger zone (CTZ). It can cause extra-pyramidal side-effects. (**Domperidone** can also be used as a motility agent. Its prokinetic effect is exerted at the oesophago-gastric and gastroduodenal junctions – it does not cross the blood–brain barrier and consequently does not have any central side-effects.)
2 **Haloperidol** blocks dopamine receptors at the CTZ. **Cyclizine** blocks histamine receptors at the VC and can be used together with haloperidol.
3 **Levomepromazine** (**methotrimeprazine**) blocks D_3, $5HT_3$, ACh and H_1 receptors. It is potentially sedating in doses greater than $6.25\,mg/24$ hours.
4 **Odansetron/granisetron** blocks $5HT_3$ centrally and peripherally.
5 Others include **octreotide**, a somatostatin analogue, and **dexamethasone**.

Complementary treatments should also be considered. Acupuncture, reflexology, aromatherapy and massage may help to relax the patient and reduce their anxiety and fear. Behaviour/aversion therapy can help to reduce the 'learnt' vomiting reflex in response to unpleasant stimuli (e.g. to the site of the chemotherapy needles or even to the chemotherapy ward).

It was decided to start Mrs Brown on a combination of haloperidol (to combat the nausea and vomiting due to opioids and tumour toxins) and cyclizine (to combat any symptoms due to ascites, hepatomegaly, hepatic disease, squashed stomach syndrome and anxiety).

Step 8 – individualise the treatment

Because of the constant vomiting it was decided to administer these drugs via a syringe driver.

Step 9 – set realistic goals for treatment

The aim of treatment was to try to eliminate nausea and reduce the frequency of vomiting to once or twice a day. Mrs Brown felt that this would bring about a vast improvement in the quality of her life.

Step 10 – assess the patient's response to treatment

Within 24 hours Mrs Brown felt remarkably better and had stopped feeling so nauseated. She continued to be sick, although infrequently.

Step 11 – review!

Over time, Mrs Brown's condition deteriorated, but her nausea and vomiting remained quite well controlled unless she was distressed. To try to reduce her anxiety, a change of anti-emetic to levomepromazine was suggested. However, when it was explained to Mrs Brown that this might make her drowsy, she refused the treatment, as staying in control and being alert were very important to her. She was then offered massage treatment, which helped her to relax and also improved her symptoms. Finally, she started to discuss some of her spiritual worries. She relaxed markedly and her vomiting improved dramatically.

Box 2.6:   Self-assessment questions

- List the common causes of nausea and vomiting.
- Draw a diagram to show how stimuli act centrally to cause nausea and vomiting.
- Which neurotransmitter receptors are involved, and how do the various anti-emetics work?
- What is the 'stepwise' treatment for nausea and vomiting?

'I can't breathe' – breathlessness

Case 2.2

Five years ago, Mrs White, aged 72 years, underwent a right mastectomy for breast cancer. She subsequently developed a swelling in her right axilla and mild lymphoedema of her right hand. This was assumed to be due to secondary lymph-node spread from her original tumour. She was treated with radiotherapy and only three cycles of chemotherapy, as this made her extremely unwell. Six months later she presented in the surgery with increasing breathlessness. Her only medication at that time was tamoxifen.

Step 1 – list of problem symptoms

Breathlessness, swollen arm, lack of energy, and anxiety.

Step 2 – prioritise the symptoms

Breathlessness (the patient could no longer go ballroom dancing).

Step 3 – list the possible causes

Box 2.7:   Possible causes of symptoms in Case 2.2

Illness
- Cancer of the bronchus
- Pleural effusion
- Lymphangitis carcinomatosa
- Superior vena cava (SVC) obstruction
- Pulmonary embolism
- Anaemia
- Pericardial effusion
- Ascites-diaphragmmatic splinting

Treatment
- Radiotherapy
- Chemotherapy agents (e.g. bleomycin)
- Other drugs (e.g. aspirin, non-steroidal anti-inflammatory drugs [NSAIDS], hormones for pulmonary emboli)
- Hickman line for pneumothorax

Other causes
- Asthma
- Chronic obstructive airways disease (COAD)
- Infection
- Cardiac causes – left ventricular failure (LVF), arrhythmias
- Anxiety/fear

Step 4 – establish the probable diagnosis

Mrs White's chest X-ray and full blood count were normal. Her spirometry showed a slightly restrictive pattern. This was thought to be due to mild chronic obstructive airways disease (COAD) caused by her previous smoking. A ventilation/perfusion (VQ) scan was performed which showed small mismatched areas. A diagnosis of mild COAD and multiple pulmonary emboli was made. In this case, the predisposing factors for pulmonary emboli were malignant disease and tamoxifen.

Box 2.8   Establishing the probable diagnosis

History

- Previous chest problems/smoker? – COAD.
- Exacerbating factors – asthma.
- Haemoptysis – bronchial carcinoma/pulmonary emboli/infection.
- Pain/palpitations – cardiac causes.
- Purulent sputum – infection.

Examination

- Appearance pink/blue – COAD.
- Lymph nodes – metastases.
- Auscultation – wheeze – space-occupying lesion (SOL)/asthma;
          – crackles – infection/fibrosis/lymphangitis carcinomatosa;
          – dullness – effusion/consolidation.

Investigation

- Full blood count, chest X-ray, spirometry, ECG, ventilation perfusion (VQ) scan.
- Arterial oxygen saturation.

Steps 5 and 6 – establish the patient's understanding of the problem and discuss possible causes

Step 7 – decide on the most relevant treatment

General measures (often the most useful approach of all)

- Sit upright.
- Reassure the patient (e.g. with familiar faces).
- Provide adequate ventilation – open window or use a fan.
- Oxygen – this often acts more as a psychological support than by improving oxygen concentration.
- Morphine – either as linctus or nebulised.
- Counselling and breathing re-training.

Specific measures

Mrs White was started on the bronchodilator salbutamol, inhaled steroids and warfarin. Her tamoxifen was changed to medroxyprogesterone acetate.

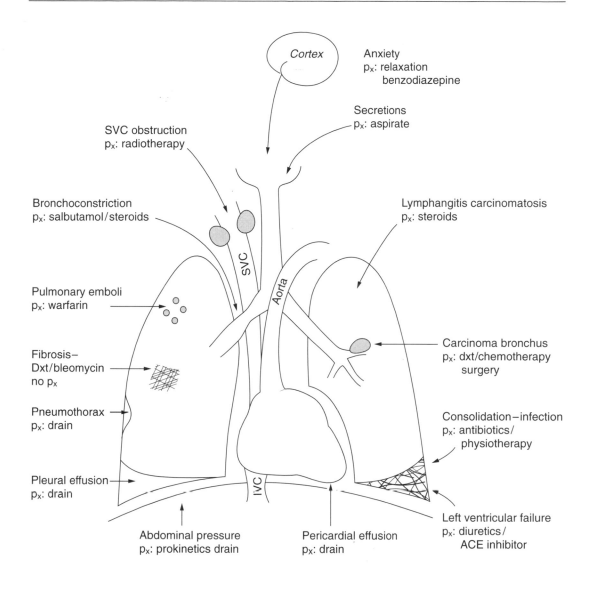

Figure 2.2 Specific causes of and treatments for dyspnoea.

> **Box 2.9: Key point**
>
> Superior vena cava (SVC) obstruction constitutes an emergency!
> Treatment with 16 mg dexamethasone should be started and an urgent radiotherapy opinion sought.

Step 8 – individualise the treatment

Step 9 – set realistic goals for treatment

Mrs White wanted to be able to ballroom dance again. After a while she came to accept that this was not going to be possible. She compromised by setting the goal of being able to walk down the road.

Step 10 – assess the patient's response to treatment

Her treatment made little difference to her symptoms.

Step 11 – review!

Mrs White continued to become increasingly breathless despite her treatment. Her distress escalated as she became more disabled by her symptoms. She was given morphine solution 10 mg prn and oxygen to use as necessary. She failed to improve, and nebulised morphine was tried,[7] with little success. Knowing that so often just having someone with the patient can help to relieve anxiety, a lot of time was spent with her. Sometimes this was to try to calm and reassure her, but at other times it was just in order to 'be there'. Mrs White was offered relaxation tapes and counselling. A small dose of diazepam, 2 mg qds prn, was started, as the risks of respiratory depression were negligible compared to the benefits of relaxing.

Despite these efforts, she failed to improve. She never accepted her deterioration or talked about the possibility that she might not get better. She was finally rushed into hospital acutely breathless, and subsequently died from bronchopneumonia.

The real reason for her continual deterioration was never established.

> **Box 2.10: Self-assessment questions**
>
> • What are the common causes of breathlessness?
> • What non-pharmacological measures can be used to alleviate breathlessness?

'I am so constipated' – constipation

Case 2.3

Mr Tucker, a 70-year-old retired farmer, has carcinoma of the prostate with bone secondaries. He has recently experienced increasing pain, and has had his dose of MST increased to 130 mg bd. His other medication includes diclofenac, 75 mg bd, for bone pain and amitriptyline, 75 mg od, for depression. He is complaining that his bowels will not work.

Step 1 – list of problem symptoms

Pain, depression and constipation.

Step 2 – prioritise the symptoms

Constipation is the greatest concern

Step 3 – list the possible causes

Box 2.11:   Possible causes of symptoms in Case 2.3

Illness
- Bowel obstruction
- Hypercalcaemia
- General debility

Treatment
- Drugs (e.g. opioids, amitriptyline)

Other causes
- Poor diet
- Decreased exercise
- Low fluid intake
- Electrolyte imbalance
- Hypothyroidism

Step 4 – establish the probable diagnosis

Box 2.12:   Establishing the probable diagnosis

History

- Is this true constipation (i.e. straining to pass hard stools)?
- How long has this been a problem?
- Is flatus being passed?

Examination

- Does the patient have a distended abdomen? Is their colon palpable?
- Rectal examination – faeces in rectum.

Investigation

- Urea and electrolytes and calcium level; thyroid function test.
- The differential diagnosis is bowel obstruction. An abdominal X-ray should show a colon packed with faeces.

Mr Tucker had a history consistent with constipation. He had a distended abdomen and a rectum loaded with hard faecal pellets. This was thought to be due to his medication (consisting of opioids and amitriptyline), his depression, his general debility and his poor diet.

Steps 5 and 6 – establish the patient's understanding of the problem and discuss possible causes

Step 7 – decide on the most relevant treatment

Specific measures

- Change the MST to a less constipating opioid (e.g. fentanyl).[8]
- Change the antidepressant.
- Increase intake of dietary fibre and fluids.

General measures

```
┌─────────────────────────────────────────────────────────────────────────┐
│ Box 2.13:   General treatment measures                                    │
│                                                                           │
│ Bulking agents        Fybogel      ⎫                                      │
│                       Normacol     ⎬  High fibre content                  │
│                       Trifyba      ⎭                                      │
│                                                                           │
│ Softeners             Lactulose       Osmotic agent, draws water into bowel│
│                       Poloxamer                                           │
│                       Docusate                                            │
│                                                                           │
│ Stimulants            Bisacodyl    ⎫                                      │
│                       Senna        ⎬                                      │
│                       Glycerine    ⎬  Also available as pessaries         │
│                       Danthron     ⎭                                      │
│                                                                           │
│ Combination drugs     Co-danthrusate     (danthron and docusate)         │
│                       Co-danthramer       (danthron and poloxamer 1:8)   │
│                       Co-danthramer forte (danthron and poloxamer 1:13)  │
│                                                                           │
│ Enemas                Microlax                                            │
│                       Phosphate                                           │
└─────────────────────────────────────────────────────────────────────────┘
```

- Anticipate problems, start prophylactic treatment early.
- Titrate the dosage against symptoms.
- Aim to use a softener/osmotic agent and stimulant.
- Fixed-dose combinations aid patient compliance but do not allow flexibility in the ratio of softener to stimulant.
- In cases of faecal impaction, use enemas.

```
┌─────────────────────────────────────────────────────────────────────────┐
│ Box 2.14:   Key points                                                    │
│                                                                           │
│ • Constipation can be more difficult to treat than pain.                  │
│ • Anticipate problems early. Start treatment prophylactically.            │
│ • To treat effectively, combine a stool softener with a bowel stimulant.  │
└─────────────────────────────────────────────────────────────────────────┘
```

Mr Tucker's diet was discussed and his fluid intake was increased. His MST was changed to fentanyl patches, 75 microgramme/hour, and his amitriptyline was changed to sertraline. Microlax enemas were used to help to empty his rectum and relieve his discomfort, and co-danthramer forte, 10 mL bd, was used to soften his stool and aid its expulsion.

Step 8 – individualise the treatment

As above, by use of liquids, capsules, and enemas as appropriate.

Step 9 – set realistic goals for treatment

The aim of treatment was to stop using enemas as soon as possible and to pass a softish stool every 2–3 days with minimal straining.

Step 10 – assess the patient's response to treatment

This improved initially.

Step 11 – review

After 10 days Mr Tucker developed uncontrollable watery diarrhoea. A rectal examination revealed a hard faecal mass impacted in his rectum. He had constipation with overflow diarrhoea. He was restarted on enemas, and his dose of co-danthramer forte was increased to 20 mL bd. His bowels settled into a regular pattern, but he remained depressed and in some pain.

Box 2.15: Key point

• Diarrhoea can be due to constipation!

Box 2.16: Self-assessment questions

• Name the different laxatives used.
• How do they work?

'I can't go to the toilet' – bowel obstruction

Case 2.4

Mrs Jones is a 62-year-old woman with extensive ovarian carcinoma. She has locally invasive tumour and hepatic and lymph node secondaries. She has become increasingly constipated and is experiencing some abdominal discomfort and nausea.

Step 1 – list of problem symptoms

Constipation, abdominal pain and nausea.

Step 2 – prioritise the symptoms

Constipation.

Step 3 – list the possible causes

For constipation, *see* Box 2.11 above.
For bowel obstruction, *see* Box 2.17.

Box 2.17:   Possible causes of symptoms in Case 2.4

Illness	• Tumour in the abdominal cavity
Treatment	• Adhesions following surgery
Other causes	• Metabolic disturbances
	• Ischaemia
	• Torsion
	• Further causes can be found in any surgical textbook

Step 4 – establish the probable diagnosis

Box 2.18:   Establishing the probable diagnosis

History

- How long has the constipation been a problem?
- Is it absolute (i.e. no faeces or flatus)?
- Is there any associated pain?
- Is there any nausea or vomiting? This may be profuse if there is a high gastric outlet obstruction.

Classical symptoms of intestinal obstruction (i.e. colicky abdominal pain, nausea and vomiting and absolute constipation) may present acutely, but more commonly in malignant obstruction they have an insiduous onset and may vary in intensity at different times.

Examination

- Classically abdominal distension with tympanitic bowel sounds. A malignant abdominal mass may be felt.

Investigations

- Endoscopy for high obstruction
- Abdominal X-ray (erect/supine), to differentiate between constipation and bowel obstruction, or if surgery is contemplated.

Mrs Jones had a 2-week history of increasing constipation, which had ended with absolute constipation over the last 5 days. She experienced nausea, vomiting and some mild colicky abdominal pains. Her abdomen was distended, but there was no localised tenderness. Bowel sounds were active with an occasional tympanitic sound. Her rectum was empty.

A clinical diagnosis of bowel obstruction was made, and no further investigations were performed.

Steps 5 and 6 – establish the patient's understanding of the problem and discuss possible causes

Mrs Jones understood that she had extensive disease. She did not want any interventive treatment, and she agreed to palliative medical treatment of her bowel obstruction.

Step 7 – decide on the most relevant treatment

Surgical management

This should be considered as an option for every patient. About 30% of cases have a non-malignant cause for their symptoms. Even when the obstruction is due to malignancy, many patients enjoy considerable symptom-free periods following palliative surgery.[9]

Box 2.19:   Key point

Always consider the option of surgery.

Medical management

- To manage abdominal pain and colic, stop all stimulant laxatives (e.g. senna) and prokinetic drugs (e.g. metaclopramide). Give diamorphine for pain and hyoscine butylbromide for colic.[9] The latter also helps to reduce the size and frequency of vomits, as it decreases gastric secretions.
- To control nausea and vomiting, *see* Case 2.1 above. The anti-emetic of choice is usually cyclizine.
- A small proportion of patients with high gastric outlet obstruction may be more comfortable with nasogastric aspiration, but this should be the exception, not the rule.
- Patients should be allowed to eat and drink as they choose.
- Dexamethasone may help to relieve symptoms if obstruction is high or due to lymphoma.

• If the symptoms are no better after 3 or 4 days, consider using the somatostatin analogue, octreotide.[8] This reduces gastric secretions and helps to reduce the volume and frequency of vomits.

Due to Mrs Jones' extensive disease and previous combination chemotherapy, surgery was not considered to be a reasonable treatment. She was therefore started on diamorphine, cyclizine and hyoscine butylbromide.

Step 8 – individualise the treatment

Once the bowel is obstructed, oral medication is unlikely to be absorbed. Drugs should therefore be given via syringe driver.

Step 9 – goals

The aim was to reduce Mrs Jones' discomfort and enable her to eat small amounts of food.

Box 2.20: Key point

Most patients with bowel obstruction due to malignancy can be managed palliatively without nasogastric suction.

Step 10 – assess the patient's response to treatment

Mrs Jones' nausea settled quickly and she became pain free. She continued to vomit occasionally.

Step 11 – review!

After 7 days Mrs Jomes' vomiting started to increase again. She was started on octreotide administered via a second syringe driver, and her symptoms improved again.

Box 2.21: Self-assessment questions

• What are the treatment options for bowel obstruction?
• How should drugs be administered? Why?

'I can't do anything' – fatigue/weakness

Case 2.5

Mrs Lewis is a 50-year-old woman with breast cancer. She has recently developed some lower thoracic back pain and has become very tired and lethargic. She feels that her memory is deteriorating.

Step 1 – list of problem symptoms

Back pain, lethargy, tiredness and loss of memory.

Step 2 – prioritise the symptoms

Tiredness.

Step 3 – list the possible causes

Box 2.22: Key point

The complaint of fatigue is so nearly universal in patients with malignant disease that it can be overlooked as a sign of serious but treatable disease.

Box 2.23: Possible causes of symptoms in Case 2.5

Illness	• Tumour load
	• Hypercalcaemia
	• Spinal cord compression
Treatment	• Drug accumulation (e.g. opioids, diazepam)
	• Radiotherapy
	• Chemotherapy
	• Steroids can cause myopathy
Other causes	• Anaemia
	• Infection

- Anxiety/depression
- Insomnia
- Anorexia
- Cardiac failure
- Respiratory failure
- Metabolic disturbance (e.g. potassium or sodium)
- Thyroid disease

Step 4 – establish the probable diagnosis

Box 2.24:   Establishing the probable diagnosis

History

- Pay great attention to this – listen to what the patient says and to how it is said, as it may well be your best clue to the diagnosis!
- What does the patient mean?
- When did it begin?
- Is the weakness localised or generalised?

Examination

To include in full the nervous system, musculoskeletal system and mental state.

Investigation

- Directed by history and examination to include full blood count, urea and electrolytes, calcium, thyroid function tests, chest X-ray, etc.

Beware of the following two conditions that can present insidiously with weakness.

Hypercalcaemia

This presents with:

- weakness;
- aching;
- nausea and vomiting;
- confusion;
- polyuria;
- constipation.

It is usually due to the production of a parathormone-like protein by the tumour, a process that is unrelated to the presence of bone metastases. A corrected calcium level of >2.8 mmol/L is abnormal[10] (check serum calcium/albumen to correct for low albumen).

Spinal cord compression

Suspect this if the patient has any of the following:

- back pain which is worse on lying;
- coughing or straining;
- if there is a sensory change (usually one or two dermatomes below the level of compression), motor weakness or sphincter disturbance.

This is an emergency situation!

Box 2.25:   Key point

Spinal cord compression is an emergency situation!

Mrs Lewis gave a history of generalised fatigue and overall weakness that had been progressing for several weeks but had deteriorated during the last 2 weeks. Examination did not reveal any obvious signs of illness. However, blood analysis did show her to be mildly anaemic (Hb 9.8 g/dL), and her corrected calcium level was raised at 3.5 mmol/L (normal range 2.2–2.6 mmol/L). A diagnosis of hypercalcaemia was made.

Steps 5 and 6 – establish the patient's understanding of the problem and discuss possible causes

Mrs Lewis had wondered whether her symptoms were due to further breast disease, or if it was all due to 'her age'. It was explained to her that it probably meant she had recurrent disease and that this would need to be investigated once her high calcium level had been corrected.

Step 7 – decide on the most relevant treatment

Specific measures

These are related to underlying pathology (e.g. antibiotics for infection, change opioid, give food supplements).

Hypercalcaemia

Initially decide whether this is a terminal event. If it is a new event, the patient's quality of life has been good, or it is a long time since the last episode – treat! Rehydrate the patient as necessary. Treat with bisphosphonates, IV pamidronate 60–90 mg in 500 ml of 0.9% saline over 4 hours.[8] Review the antitumour treatment. Monitor for recurrence – check the calcium level after 3 days if the symptoms have not improved significantly, or every 2 weeks if the treatment appears to be successful.

Spinal cord compression

Start treatment urgently. Give dexamethasone, either 24 mg IV over 2 minutes if symptoms have been present for less than 1 week, or 18 mg orally if deterioration has been slower. Arrange immediately to see an oncologist for a definitive diagnosis (i.e. MRI scan) and treatment (either surgery or radiotherapy).

Non-specific measures

If increased tumour load is suspected as a cause of weakness, consider giving dexamethasone 4 mg o.d. Stop after 1 week if there is no benefit. Maintain the drug at this level if it is beneficial, unless the patient has a long-term prognosis of several months, in which case attempt to reduce the dose to 2 mg o.d. Medroxyprogesterone acetate, 400 mg daily, may also be worth trying to stimulate the patient's appetite and encourage weight gain.[10]

Mrs Lewis was rehydrated with 3 L of normal saline over a period of 36 hours, and then received a pamidronate infusion.

Step 8 – individualise the treatment

The decision to treat the specific causes of fatigue and weakness must be weighed up carefully. Are these symptoms of terminal illness?

In Mrs Lewis's case her deterioration had been rapid, her quality of life had been good, and this was her first episode of hypercalcaemia. The decision to treat was an easy one!

Step 9 – set realistic goals for treatment

The aim of treatment was to restore the ionised calcium level to normal, and to improve the symptoms of fatigue, weakness and memory loss.

Step 10 – assess the patient's response to treatment

Mrs Lewis's calcium level dropped to below 2.8 mmol/L. She felt much better, stronger and more energetic, and her memory improved.

Step 11 – review!

Mrs Lewis was due to be fully assessed with a chest X-ray, CT scan and bone scan to try to locate the site of her recurrent tumour. While she was waiting for these investigations she became aware of increasing pain in her back and numbness in her feet. She had gone home for a few days, and telephoned her community nurse to ask for some incontinence pads as she had developed a dribbling incontinence. The doctor also visited that day and recognised the signs of an acute spinal cord compression. Dexamethasone, 18 mg orally, was started immediately and Mrs Lewis was rushed to the oncology centre. An MRI scan detected a compression at the level of the tenth and eleventh thoracic vertebrae, and radiotherapy was started within 12 hours of the diagnosis being made at home. Prompt action managed to save Mrs Lewis from paraplegia.

Box 2.26:   Key point

Beware of the patient with fatigue, weakness of legs, back pain and sudden onset of urinary incontinence!

Box 2.27:   Self-assessment questions

- List the common causes of weakness and fatigue.
- Name two important conditions that can present insidiously in this way.
- How do they present and how should you treat them?

'He seems so muddled' – confusion

Case 2.6

Mr James is 56 years old and has disseminated colon cancer with known hepatic secondaries. He is jaundiced and itchy. His wife, who is caring for him at home, contacts their GP in great distress as her husband has become very confused and she woke in the night and found him trying to get out of the front door to go to work.

Step 1 – list of problem symptoms

Confusion with disorientation in time and possibly place, jaundice and itching. His wife's distress should also be considered.

Step 2 – prioritise the symptoms

Confusion.

Step 3 – list the possible causes

Box 2.28:   Possible causes of symptoms in Case 2.6

Illness	• Cerebral tumour (primary or secondary) • Hypercalcaemia
Treatment	• Drugs (e.g. opioids, corticosteroids)
Other causes	• Biochemical abnormality (e.g. uraemia, liver dysfunction) • Infection • Recent trauma • Alcohol withdrawal • Cardiac failure • Respiratory failure

---

Step 4 – establish the probable diagnosis

Box 2.29:   Establishing the probable diagnosis

History

- Is it of recent onset? Suggests acute confusional state.
- Fluctuating course, disorganised thought, inattention, memory impairment and disorientation suggests acute confusion.
- Longer history, less symptom fluctuation and unchanged alertness suggests possible dementia.

Examination

- Relate to possible physical causes (e.g. chest examination, etc.).
- Perform full CNS and mental health assessment.

Investigation

- According to physical findings (e.g. blood cultures, chest auscultation, etc., skull X-ray, MRI scan, etc.).

Mr James had become confused over a period of 3–4 days. His confusion seemed to vary throughout the day, and was particularly distressing at night, when he became far more restless and often wandered round the house. His medication had recently been increased from MST 200 mg bd to 300 mg bd, together with metoclopramide, 10 mg qds prn, co-danthramer, 10 mL bd, and temazepam, 20 mg at night. He had also been started on dexamethasone, 4 mg daily, 5 days earlier to try to reduce discomfort due to liver capsule stretch and to decrease his itching. Examination found him slightly jaundiced, with a hard palpable liver edge. His chest was clear on auscultation, and there were no other signs of infection. Central nervous system examination, including fundoscopy, was normal. Blood examination revealed a mild anaemia. Hepatic function was impaired, with a bilirubin level of 121 mmol/L (normal range <17 mmol/l). An alkaline phosphatase level of 710 IU/L (normal range 20–130 IU/L) and lactate dehydrogenase (LDH) level of 2700 IU/L (normal range < 500 IU/L) were found. His calcium level (corrected for albumen level) was normal, as were his urea and electrolyte levels.

Mr James' confusion was diagnosed as being due to hepatic failure, possibly exacerbated by opioid treatment.

Steps 5 and 6 – establish the patient's understanding of the problem and discuss possible causes

Most of the discussion took place with Mrs James. She understood that her husband was seriously ill. It was explained to her that his confusion was probably a sign of terminal disease, and that the aim of treatment would be to try to alleviate her husband's distress and anxiety.

Step 7 – decide on the most relevant treatment

Specific measures

- Treat specific causes (e.g. antibiotics for infection, reduce calcium levels if raised).
- Alter any possible exacerbating drugs if possible (e.g. dexamethasone).

General measures

- Maintain familiar faces and surroundings.
- Maintain a light quiet environment.
- Keep to a steady routine.

Drugs

- Thioridazine, 25 mg stat., then 10–25 mg tds according to the response. This is most suitable for the elderly, or in patients who are only mildly confused.
- Haloperidol, 0.5–5 mg orally or subcutaneously stat., then tds, or hourly for two more doses until settled. This is most appropriate for the more confused, psychotic patient.
- Levomepromazine, 25–50 mg subcutaneously stat. if more sedation is required.
- Midazolam, 2–10 mg subcutaneously, or diazepam PR if the patient is acutely confused but not psychotic and sedation is required.

General measures were looked at to help Mr James. His dexamethasone was stopped and he was started on 5 mg haloperidol at night.

Step 8 – individualise the treatment

The haloperidol was given orally, as Mr James was not experiencing any difficulty with swallowing and was willing to take medication.

Step 9 – set realistic goals for treatment

The aim was to achieve more peaceful nights so that Mrs James could sleep, and hopefully she would be able to maintain her husband's care at home.

Step 10 – assess the patient's response to treatment

Mr James still had periods of confusion, but he seemed less distressed by them and slept better.

Step 11 – review!

Over the following days Mr James became weaker and drowsier. His medication was switched to administration via syringe driver, and he subsequently died peacefully at home.

Box 2.30:   Self-assessment questions

- How can one tell the difference between acute and chronic confusional states?
- What non-medical measures can be implemented as treatment?
- What pharmacological treatments can be used to help with confusional states?
- Which patients do they benefit?

Other common symptoms

The final section of this chapter consists of a brief discussion of some other symptoms. It is not comprehensive, but covers a few salient points about each symptom and its possible management.

Depression

This is probably seen in up to a one-third of patients. The way in which the bad news about the patient's diagnosis and prognosis is given may play a significant part in determining who develops depression (P. Maguire, personal communication).

Consider whether the patient is quiet, withdrawn, tearful, waking early, anorexic, feeling that life is worthless or feeling suicidal.

Treat with tricyclics or selective serotonin reuptake inhibitors (SSRIs). The two groups of antidepressants are equally effective. The increased level of side-effects and risk of fatality in overdose with tricyclics will need to be balanced against the cost of SSRIs.

Urinary symptoms

Symptoms include frequency and urgency, hesitancy and retention, spasms and incontinence.

Treatments include the following:

- infection – antibiotic;
- urgency – amitriptyline/imipramine/oxybutynin;
- hesitancy – indoramin/bethanacol;
- spasms – consider amitriptyline/oxybutynin, monitor for infection, change catheter balloon size or catheter.

Hiccups

These may be due to gastric distension, diaphragmatic irritation, uraemia, infection or a CNS tumour.

Treatments include the following:

- rub the palate as far back as possible;
- decrease gastric distension (e.g. with peppermint water, asilone, metaclopramide);
- relax muscle (e.g. with baclofen, nifedipine, midazolam);
- central inhibition (e.g. with haloperidol, chlorpromazine).

Pruritus

This may be due to uraemia, bile salts, skin disease, drugs (e.g. opioids), thyroid disease, myeloma, lymphoma or polycythaemia rubra vera.
   Treatments include the following:

- simple measures such as use of a moisturiser, cooler shorter baths, and avoiding the use of additives in bath water (e.g. bubble bath);
- drug treatments, including antihistamines and dexamethasone or stanozolol for cholestatic jaundice.

Terminal rattle

This is due to secretions collecting in the pharynx.

- Ensure that the patient is not distressed.
- Try to reposition the patient.
- Explain the problem to the relatives – they are often more distressed than the patient.
- Consider giving glycopyrronium or hyoscine hydrobromide. This may need to be repeated.
- If the patient is deeply unconscious, try suction.

Ascites

- Treat the condition if it is causing discomfort, vomiting or dyspnoea.
- Diuretics (e.g. frusemide or spironolactone) may be tried, but paracentesis is usually necessary. If the prognosis is extended, consider a shunt which drains the ascitic fluid back into the venous system.

Flushes/sweats

These may be due to hormonal manipulation, chemotherapy, radiotherapy, tumour (usually with hepatic secondaries), infection, myeloma or drugs (e.g. opioids).

- Treat specific causes. If there is pyrexia with sweats, use non-steroidal anti-inflammatory drugs (NSAIDs). If there is no pyrexia, consider thioridazine or propantheline.

Conclusion

The condition of patients is constantly changing, and just as one problem may seem to have improved another one may appear. For patients in the terminal phase of their illness such change can occur with frightening rapidity. Be aware of this, and at every patient contact remember to Review, Review and Review!

Remember also that patients are first and foremost individuals with their own healthcare beliefs, fears and ideas. Listen to them and give them time – they have so much to tell us!

References

1   World Health Organisation (1990) *Cancer Pain Relief and Palliative Care*. Technical Report Series 804. World Health Organisation, Geneva.

2   Donnelly S and Walsh D (1995) The symptoms of advanced cancer. *Semin Oncol.* **22**: 67–72.

3   Buckman R (1994) *How to Break Bad News*. Pan, London.

4   Links M and Kramer J (1994) Breaking bad news: realistic versus unrealistic hopes. *Support Cancer Care.* **2**: 91–3.

5   Lichter I (1993) Which antiemetic? *J Palliative Care.* **9**: 42–50.

6   Twycross R and Back I (1998) Nausea and vomiting in advanced cancer. *Eur J Palliative Care.* **5**: 39–44.

7   Lydford Davis C (1994) The therapeutics of dyspnoea. *Cancer Surveys Vol. 21. Palliative Medicine: Problem Areas in Pain and Symptom Management.* Imperial Cancer Research Fund, London.

8   Twycross R, Wilcock A and Thorp S (1998) *PCF1 Palliative Care Formulary*. Radcliffe Medical Press, Oxford.

9   Baines M (1995) The pathophysiology and management of malignant intestinal obstruction. In D Doyle, G Hanks and N Macdonald (eds) *Oxford Textbook of Palliative Medicine*. Oxford Medical Publications, Oxford.

10 Regnard CFB and Tempest S (1998) *A Guide to Symptom Relief in Advanced Disease*. Hochland and Hochland, Manchester.

To learn more

Doyle D, Hanks G and Macdonald N (1995) *Oxford Textbook of Palliative Medicine*. Oxford Medical Publications, Oxford.

Regnard CFB and Tempest S (1998) *A Guide to Symptom Relief in Advanced Disease* (4e). Hochland and Hochland, Manchester.

Twycross R (1999) *Introducing Palliative Care* (3e). Radcliffe Medical Press, Oxford.

Twycross R, Wilcock A and Thorp S (1998) *PCF1 Palliative Care Formulary*. Radcliffe Medical Press, Oxford.

CHAPTER 3

Continuous subcutaneous infusion

Jo Cooper and Trevor Mitten

What is a syringe driver

A syringe-driver is a power-driven device that holds a prepared syringe. Working on a pre-set timer, the power-driven device pushes the syringe plunger forward to administer accurately controlled amounts of a drug.

The MS16^A and MS26 are battery-powered ambulatory syringe drivers which can be carried by the patient during treatment, without interfering unduly with the normal activities of daily living. The differences between the MS16^A and MS26 are listed in Table 3.1.

Table 3.1 Differences between the MS16^A and MS26 syringe drivers

- The MS16^A has a *BLUE* label
- The MS26 has a *GREEN* label

	MS16^A hourly rate	*MS26 daily rate*
Rate range	0–99 mm *per hour*	0–99 mm *per 24 hours*
Indicator light flashes	Every second	Every 25 seconds
Boost	No	Yes
Label colour	Blue	Green

Differences in driver use

- The MS16^A rate is set in millimetres (mm) *per hour* with a typical infusion range of 30 minutes to 60 hours. It has a variable speed of 0–99 mm per hour.
- The MS26 rate is set in millimetres (mm) *per day* with a typical infusion range of 12 hours to 60 days. It has a variable speed of 0–99 mm per day with a bolus of 0.23 mm of travel.

Battery life

The battery life for both syringe drivers is 50 full syringes.

Alarm sounds

The alarm sounds are as follows:

- end of travel – an audible alarm sounds and the pump stops;
- occlusion – an audible alarm sounds and the pump stops;
- low battery – the indicator light stops flashing.

Figures 3.1, 3.2 and 3.3 illustrate the visual differences between the two types of syringe driver.

How to use the syringe driver

The following list of **Do's** and **Dont's** may be helpful when considering the use of the syringe driver.

Do's

- Do check the battery daily and maintain regular service intervals.
- Do give the patient and their relative(s) a clear verbal explanation *and* written guidelines.
- Do check both verbally and visually to ensure that the patient and their relative(s) understand the equipment and its use.

Dont's

- Don't get the syringe driver wet. It is not waterproof and the dampness will affect the performance or the equipment, or both.

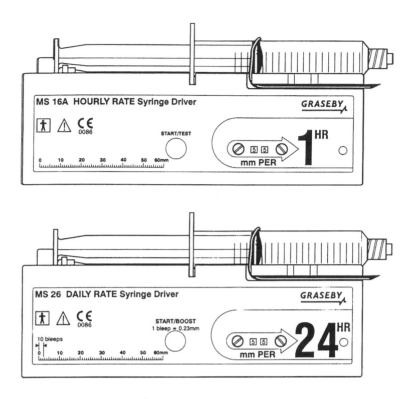

Figure 3.1   Differences between MS16^A and MS26 syringe drivers.

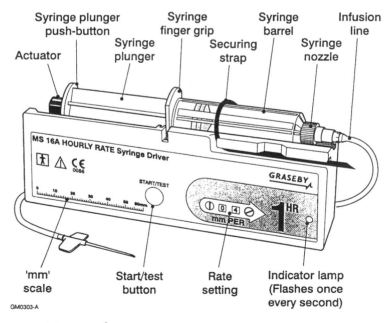

Figure 3.2   Features of the MS16^A syringe driver.

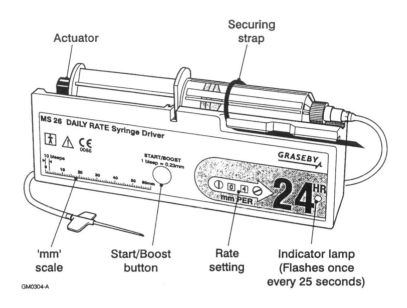

Figure 3.3 Features of the MS26 syringe driver.

- Don't open it up to look inside. This will damage the equipment and affect its performance.
- Don't wipe the syringe driver with organic cleansing solvents or strong disinfectant.
- Don't use mobile phones close to the equipment.

Why use a syringe driver

There are times when it is appropriate for medication to be given via the subcutaneous route.[1] The principal indicators for the use of the syringe driver include the following:

- the patient being unable to take oral medication.
- dysphagia;
- severe weakness;
- pain control;
- nausea and vomiting;
- unconsciousness.

Continuous subcutaneous infusions take a while to work. It will take some time for the syringe-driver medication to reach optimum plasma levels. Therefore it is important to adopt other pain relief measures until the patient feels the effect of the infusion. This is referred to as a *loading dose* of medication.[2] It is recommended that, prior to setting up the syringe driver, subcutaneous or intramuscular medication is given.[2] This gives the patient much-needed relief of pain or symptoms while a reservoir of the drug is building up subcutaneously.

The use of continuous subcutaneous infusions provides constant medication with no peaks or troughs, and it avoids the need for repeated injections.

What is needed for subcutaneous infusion?

The following will be required when setting up the MS16[A] and MS26 subcutaneous syringe drivers:

- a 9-volt alkaline battery;
- a syringe-driver cover;
- a holster or 'bum-bag,' for mobile patients;
- a rate-adjusting key;
- a syringe;
- an infusion set;
- clear film dressing;
- diluent if required;
- the medication prescribed.

Setting up the syringe driver

The following steps should be taken when setting up the subcutaneous infusion.

- Explain to the patient and their relative(s) what you are going to do. Ensure that their consent is obtained and that they understand the advantages of the treatment before continuing with it. Do not rush your explanations.
- Choose an area of skin where there is no damage or oedema. Useful sites include the chest, abdomen, upper arm, thighs and back (useful if the patient is confused – this will avoid the line being pulled out).
- Fill the syringe with the required volume of medication. Allow for the small volume needed to prime the line.
- Connect and fill the infusion line. Ensure that all air is expelled.
- Measure the fluid length in the syringe, using the millimetre scale on the front of the syringe driver.
- Divide this distance, measured in millimetres, by the infusion time in *hours* for the MS16[A] syringe driver and in *days* for the MS26 syringe driver.
- Set the rate on the rate dials.
- Watch for drug precipitation, as this can block the needle.
- Most drugs should be mixed with water for injection rather than sodium chloride solution. This helps to prevent precipitation, but there are exceptions. If in doubt, and also for guidance, contact the local pharmacist.

- The butterfly needle with tubing should be primed with the contents of the syringe and inserted at an angle of 45 degrees into subcutaneous tissue.
- Loop the tubing around the site and secure it with a film dressing.
- Insert the syringe into the driver. The syringe should be clamped with the strap over the barrel of the syringe.
- Slide the actuator firmly against the plunger of the syringe.
- Press the start button. The light will flash.
- Put the syringe driver in its case.
- Check that the patient is comfortable, then reassess the patient's and relative's understanding of the treatment and the anticipated outcome.

Administration of the continuous subcutaneous infusion

Establish procedures for regular checks on the progress and administration of the continuous subcutaneous infusion.

The patient and their relative(s) should have awareness and understanding of the use of the syringe driver and be able to carry out a few checks to see whether:

- the volume (medication) is being delivered as expected;
- the rate is set correctly;
- the indicator light is flashing;
- the syringe driver is in good condition;
- the symptoms are being alleviated and/or controlled.

The boost facility on the MS26 syringe driver

On the MS26 syringe driver, the start/boost button can be pressed to administer a small bolus dose of medication. The syringe driver emits a bleep when a dose of medication is administered. With each bleep, the syringe plunger moves forward a controlled distance of 0.23 mm. To calculate the dose given, the following method is used.

- If the boost facility is pressed on four consecutive occasions, the plunger will move 4×0.23 mm $= 0.92$ mm – the medication administered is equal to 1 mg.

It is important to remember that for every millimetre (mm) the plunger moves forward by boosting, the time to complete the administration of the medication is shortened. This can be calculated thus: $1/48$ mm $\times$ 24 hours $= 30$ minutes.

Useful tip

If boost doses are to be used, allow extra volume in the syringe.

In the community, teaching the patient's relative(s) how to use the boost button can help to give them a sense of control when the patient is experiencing pain. In simple yet meaningful terms, they feel that they can contribute to the care of the individual, thus relieving the sense of hopelessness often experienced by relatives in such situations.

Caution

It is important to note that boosting the pump only delivers a *small amount* of the medication. This may be insufficient to control or alleviate symptoms adequately. If the patient experiences breakthrough pain, rescue-dose medication is recommended. This can be given orally, or if the patient is unable to swallow, it can be administered subcutaneously.

Drugs used in syringe drivers

The drugs that can be used for continuous subcutaneous infusion, using the MS16[A] and MS26 syringe driver, are listed in Table 3.2.

Syringes

It is helpful to use a Luer-Lock syringe. This helps to prevent the lines from becoming disconnected. The Graseby syringe drivers will hold syringe sizes from 2 mL to 35 mL. A 50-mL syringe can be used in an in-patient facility where regular observation is the norm. However, the protective cover will not fit over this size of syringe. Therefore it is important to observe regularly in case the barrel of the syringe becomes displaced.

Case 3.1

A sportsman 6 feet 5 inches tall and weighing 16 stone needed syringe driver-medication to control agitation and seizures related to his primary glioblastoma. His need for midazolam increased until eventually he was prescribed 280 mg of midazolam every 24 hours. The symptoms were well controlled on this dose, but a 50-mL syringe, changed every 8 hours, was required to achieve the infusion.

Metal reaction

Occasionally, a patient may be allergic to the metal in the cannula and develop a local tissue reaction.[3] In such cases, a Teflon-coated cannula may be used. If a

Table 3.2 Commonly used drugs in palliative care – syringe drivers

Drug	Suggested start dose over 24 hours	Suggested uses	Common side-effects	Stat. dose	Other beneficial effects
Pain					
Diamorphine	5–10 mg opioid naive	Severe pain. Only available in the UK and Canada	Constipation, sedation, confusion, nausea and vomiting	24-hour dose divided by six, or 5–10 mg, whichever is greater	Relaxation, cardiac output improved
Ketorolac	60–90 mg	Opioid-resistant bone pain	Gastric irritation	20–30 mg	Analgesic properties
Nausea and vomiting					
Cyclizine hydrochloride	50–150 mg	Established nausea. No identifiable cause. Raised intracranial pressure	Blurred vision, sedation	25–50 mg	Balance disorders
Haloperidol	5–10 mg	Opioid-induced nausea. Hallucinations, paranoia	Extra-pyramidal side-effects	1.5–5 mg	Anxiolytic. Antipsychotic in higher doses (10–20 mg)
Hyoscine hydro-bromide	800 microgramme–2 mg	Anti-secretory. Noisy breathing	Blurred vision, sedation, tachycardia	400–800 microgramme	Has anti-emetic effect
Metoclopramide	30–100 mg	Delayed gastric emptying	Extra-pyramidal side-effects	10–20 mg	
Ondansetron	8–16 mg	After chemotherapy. If other anti-emetics fail	Headache and constipation	4–8 mg	
Levomepromazine	6.25–25 mg	Refractory nausea/vomiting. Not first-line anti-emetic. Useful in cases where other anti-emetics fail	Strong sedation	12.5–25 mg	Also anxiolytic in terminal phase (75–200 mg). Analgesic properties
Octreotide	300–600 microgramme	Intestinal obstruction carcinoid syndrome. To reduce large-volume vomit	Insulin/oral hypoglycaemic dosage may need reducing, as it is potentiated. Dry mouth	100 microgramme	Carcinoid – antihormonal. Obstruction – reduces gut secretion and bowel motility
Anxiolytic					
Midazolam	10–30 mg	Terminal agitation. Anticonvulsant	Sedation	5–10 mg	Retrograde amnesia is a feature
Corticosteroid					
Dexamethasone	6–24 mg	Anti-inflammatory. Raised intracranial pressure	See Chapter 1	4–8 mg	Mix with caution to avoid precipitation. Seek pharmacy advice
Bowel Obstruction					
Hyoscine butylbromide (Buscopan)	60–120 mg	When sedation is not wanted. Good for colicky pain. Does not cross the blood–brain barrier	Dry mouth, urinary retention	20 mg	Reduces volume of vomits

Teflon-coated cannula is ineffective, rotating the site daily may help. Applying hydro-cortisone cream around the site is another useful alternative.

Skin irritation

Some drugs, such as cyclizine hydrochloride or levomepromazine, may cause skin irritation if used in high concentrations. This can be helped by:

- increasing the diluent in the syringe driver and using a larger syringe;
- changing the syringe driver 12-hourly instead of 24-hourly;
- adding hydrocortisone sodium succinate, 25–50 mg to the syringe contents to help to reduce the inflammation.[4]

Calculating the flow rate

MS16^A Blue

When using the MS16^A 'Blue', dilute the drug until the fluid length is equal to 48 mm (this will be 8 mL on a 10-mL BD syringe). Divide the fluid length by the number of hours (e.g. 48 mm/24 hours = 2 mm; rate = 2).

MS26 Green

When using the MS26 'Green', dilute the drug until the fluid length is equal to 50 mm (this will be 8 mL on a 10-mL BD syringe). Divide the fluid length by the number of days (e.g. 50 mm/1 day = 50 mm; rate = 50).

Monitoring the patient's condition

It is important that the patient and their relative(s) understand the need for the syringe driver, and the benefits that it can provide. It may be helpful to mention the use of a syringe driver early in discussions relating to possible future care needs, and to show the equipment that will be needed. This helps to allay some of the fears and concerns of the patient and relative(s), reduces anxiety and eliminates any last-minute surprises. The patient and relative(s) should always be given emergency contact details.

Regular assessment and review of medication is pivotal to good symptom control. Escalating pain requires a rapid response. This may mean changing medication more than once in a 24-hour period. Alternatively, pain may diminish following radio-therapy or chemotherapy, and consequently will need appropriate intervention.

Remember

Throughout continuous subcutaneous infusion, and indeed whenever you are in the palliative care environment, it is essential to remember the following:

- ongoing assessment;
- ongoing review;
- ongoing reassurance;
- ongoing guidance.

Finally, always attempt to be calm and confident in your approach. The patient and relative(s) look to the community professional for information and advice. If you are in doubt, ask. There is no harm in saying 'I can find that out for you'.

These are all prerequisites for effective intervention and a good clinical outcome for the patient and their relative(s).

Acknowledgement

The line drawings and some information relating to the administration of continuous subcutaneous infusion were kindly supplied by and with permission from Graseby Sims, Instruction Manual, Sims Graseby Ltd, Colonial Way, Watford WD2 4LG, UK.

Chapter 3: Questions

1 What is a syringe driver?
2 Which type of syringe driver is set using the hourly rate?
3 Which type of syringe driver is set using the daily rate?
4 What are the principal indications for the use of a syringe driver?
5 Name three appropriate areas on the body where the needle can be sited.
6 What simple checks can be made to assess whether the syringe driver is functioning correctly?

References

1   Oliver DJ (1985) The use of the syringe driver in terminal care. *Br J Clin Pharmacol.* **20**: 515–16.

2   Twycross RG and Lack SA (1983) *Symptom Control in Far Advanced Cancer: Pain Relief.* Pitman, London.

3   Palmer N (1988) Controlling breakthrough pain in palliative care. *Nurs Standard.* **13**: 53–4.

4   Twycross R (1997) *Symptom Management in Advanced Cancer* (2e). Radcliffe Medical Press, Oxford.

To learn more

Twycross R (1997) *Symptom Management in Advanced Cancer* (2e). Radcliffe Medical Press, Oxford.

Twycross R, Wilcock A and Thorpe S (1998) *PCF1 Palliative Care Formulary*. Radcliffe Medical Press, Oxford.

Chapter 3:   Answers

1 A power-driven device for pushing a syringe plunger forward to administer an accurately controlled dose of medication subcutaneously.
2 The MS16[A].
3 The MS26.
4 Inability to take oral medication, dysphagia, severe weakness, pain control, nausea and vomiting, or unconscious patient.
5 Chest, abdomen, upper arm, back or thighs.
6 The following checks can be made:

- that the volume is being delivered as expected;
- that the rate is set correctly;
- that the indicator light is flashing;
- that the syringe driver is in good condition;
- evaluation of the control of symptoms.

CHAPTER 4

Mouthcare

Elizabeth Potter

Pre-reading exercise

Before commencing this chapter, use these questions to test your knowledge of oral health.
Answers can be found at the end of the chapter.

1 What is xerostomia?
2 List five causes of poor oral health in palliative care patients.
3 A patient is complaining of a sore mouth. List three possible reasons for this.
4 Name three items of equipment you should have in order to perform an oral assessment.
5 Name three qualities of life that are affected by a sore, dirty, dry mouth.

Introduction

There can be nothing worse than having a dry, dirty and sore mouth. It can impinge upon the true essence of quality of life. Despite this, mouthcare is frequently a neglected and undervalued aspect of care. It is often treated as a poor relation to symptoms such as pain, nausea and dyspnoea.[1,2]

Oral problems with palliative patients are significant enough to warrant a much-needed change of response among those responsible for providing relief from symptoms. Many patients are immunosuppressed, malnourished and generally debilitated.[3] This results in a high level of manifestation of oral problems, which is illustrated in Box 4.1, in studies performed in a hospice environment.

Box 4.1:   Oral symptoms encountered in palliative care

Xerostomia (dry mouth) (67%)
Oral mucosal disease (82%)
Oral candidosis[4] (85%)

Disturbance of taste (26%)
Dysphagia (37%)
Soreness (42%)
Denture problems[5] (71%)

Effects of poor oral health on the palliative care patient

Oral care for the palliative patient in the community must not be overlooked. The community professional must remember that achieving symptom relief for the patient and their family is at the very heart of providing some quality of life. Poor oral health will affect the patient's ability to speak, smile, laugh, kiss, sing, and taste and enjoy food; all of these are critical social activities. Thus poor oral health may not only affect the patient but also have a major effect on the patient's relationship with others.

Definition of good mouthcare and its aim

The principal objectives of mouthcare for the patient who is very ill are as follows:

- to maintain comfort;
- to maintain cleanliness;
- to maintain moisture;
- to prevent infection.[6,7]

A healthy mouth depends on several factors:[8]

- adequate nutrition and hydration;
- a flow of saliva (see Box 4.2);
- proper functioning of the chewing apparatus;
- mechanical, regular cleansing of the oral cavity.

In the palliative patient, there are many possible reasons for interruption of these vital processes, and the community professional should be alert to them (see Box 4.3) Neglect of oral hygiene results in the fermentation of plaque, and this can occur rapidly in a dying patient. This build-up of plaque can lead to inflammation and irritation of the mouth surfaces and, if left untreated, may lead to the development of

---

Box 4.2:   Some wonders of saliva!

1 It moistens and lubricates food, and aids bolus formation.
2 It cleanses the mouth and teeth of cellular debris.
3 Lysozymes present in saliva help to control and destroy bacteria.
4 Saliva produces a neutral pH, which prevents cavity formation in teeth.
5 It acts as a solvent in which food molecules can be dissolved and thus tasted.[9]

---

infection and breakdown of the oral mucosal lining.[10] The oral cavity is composed of a mucosal lining of non-keratinised squamous epithelium, which regenerates rapidly every 7–14 days due to the constant trauma to which it is subjected.[7,11] It is due to its short cellular life that the oral mucosa is sensitive to chemotherapy and radiation treatment.[12]

Box 4.3:   Causes of poor oral health in palliative care patients

Malnutrition, dehydration and deficiency of iron, protein, and vitamins B and C[7,10,12,13]
Cytotoxic chemotherapy[7,10,11,14,15]
Radiotherapy[12–16]
Myelosuppressed or otherwise immunocompromised patients[13]
Surgery to the mouth[13]
Local tumours[15]
Antibiotic therapy[13]
Anxiety, depression and pain[12]
Oxygen therapy[12]

Think 'why'? And find out!

When visiting the patient with oral problems, it may help to focus on the following four steps:

1 What are the symptoms?
2 Why is the patient having the problem?
3 What might be the cause?
4 Perform an oral examination and assessment.

Oral assessment

Oral assessment has been identified as an essential component of effective and appropriate care in oral health.[7,17,18] For the community professional, a full oral assessment should be performed during the first encounter with the patient. This will provide a baseline or a point from which to begin renewing oral health. However, it should not be forgotten that this is an ongoing process, performed constantly and regularly to monitor the patient's response to therapy and to identify any new problems.[10] Ideally, it should be performed by the same health professional in order to avoid subjectivity.

Before beginning, remember to wash your hands, put on gloves and remove any dental appliances. Always have a working pen torch available, a tongue depressor and, if possible, a dental mirror. A full examination and assessment of the patient's oral cavity must be made, and can be scored according to findings.

Frequency of care can thus be determined according to the final score. An example of an oral assessment guide is included in Box 4.4. This has been developed for use in patients with head and neck cancer, having been adapted from previous studies,[19,20] and it may also be useful for the palliative community setting.

For the palliative patient at home, a mouthcare treatment regime conducted at not less than 3–4-hourly intervals is recommended[21,22] to reduce the potential risk of infection by micro-organisms. The frequency of mouthcare should be increased to 2-hourly intervals to reduce oral complications and maintain patient comfort,[23] and should be hourly if the patient is unconscious, mouth-breathing or receiving oxygen (which should always be humidified), or in cases where oral infection is involved, to obtain maximum comfort and cleanliness.[20]

Patient and family involvement

The patient may be experiencing anxiety, feelings of low self-esteem and loss of control. Involvement in their own care through information and education will encourage their feelings of self-worth and confidence.[10] The involvement of significant others in the patient's care should also be encouraged, and may be necessary for the management of oral health at home. Involving the patient's family can have a positive outcome, as it can reduce their sense of isolation and powerlessness when caring for their loved one.[24] However, the professional must be sensitive to the needs of family and friends who should not feel obliged to take part in mouthcare, particularly if they find the idea unappealing.

A gentle approach

Mouth treatment is a very personal concern, especially when it is being handled by another person. Consent should be obtained from the patient, and a gentle, careful and respectful approach must be employed.

Box 4.4:   Oral assessment guide

PATIENT NAME: UNIT NUMBER:

	Date:									
	Time:									
	Assessing Nurse:									
Voice 1 = normal 2 = deeper/raspy 3 = difficult/painful speech										
Swallow 1 = normal swallow 2 = painful 3 = unable to swallow										
Taste 1 = normal 2 = impaired/changed 3 = no taste										
Non-verbal communication (smiling/grimacing) 1 = normal 2 = difficult 3 = impossible										
Lips 1 = smooth, pink, moist 2 = dry/cracked 3 = ulcerated/bleeding										
Tongue 1 = pink and moist, papillae present 2 = coated or loss of papillae 3 = blistered/cracked										
Saliva 1 = watery 2 = thick or ropy 3 = absent										
Mucous membranes 1 = pink and moist 2 = reddened/coated 3 = ulcerations with or without bleeding										
Gums 1 = pink and firm 2 = oedematous, with or without redness										
Teeth/dentures 1 = clean, no debris 2 = localised plaque/debris 3 = generalised plaque/debris										
Candida 0 = No 2 = Yes										
Pain 0 = No pain 1 = Mild pain 2 = Moderate pain 3 = Severe pain										
ORAL CAVITY TOTAL SCORE										
Total score 9 or below – perform mouthcare every 3 to 4 hours. Total score 10–14 – perform mouthcare every 2 hours. Total score 15 or more – perform mouthcare every hour										

Frequent and regular care

Following a thorough assessment, the professional must decide which mouthcare regime is required and what agents to use. However, it must be remembered that the most important ingredient of oral care management is the frequency and thoroughness of care given.[22] The patient may require mouthcare even when asleep, especially in view of the fact that less saliva is produced during sleep, so providing less defence against infection.[12] However, this requires careful consideration by the carer when planning care.

Tools for providing oral care

Toothbrush

This provides an effective means of cleaning teeth and removing plaque and debris.[6,7,17,25,26] A small, soft, round-ended paediatric toothbrush is recommended, which can be purchased at any chemist or supermarket. All tooth surfaces should be brushed, and a thick tongue coating can also be gently brushed if the tongue is not too sore.

Foam sticks

This can be used if the patient's condition prevents the use of a toothbrush – for example, if spontaneous bleeding or pain is present. Foam sticks will not effeciently remove plaque,[27] but are effective in removing thick mucus and food debris from the mouth.

From my own practical experience, the ideal approach would be to use both tools together, as they appear to complement each other in their use.

Toothpaste

This must contain fluoride to prevent cavity formation.[7] Toothpaste is inexpensive, refreshing and effective in removing plaque as long as the brushing technique is thorough.[12] Patients should use whichever brand they prefer, but for those with sensitive teeth a paste containing strontium chloride (i.e. Sensodyne) can prevent painful stimuli from reaching exposed nerves.[7,12] It must be remembered that thorough rinsing afterwards to remove all toothpaste is important, and that the toothpaste does not cause any burning of delicate oral mucosa.[12]

Cleansing agents

Warm saline mouthwashes

This is generally recommended.[12,20] Saline is thought to promote healing and the formation of granulation tissue.[28] It is widely available and relatively pleasant to use. It has also been suggested that an agent that is soothing and does not cause pain is more likely to be used regularly by the patient.[20] Saline mouthwashes can also be made up at home using 5 mL (1 teaspoonful) of salt to 500 mL (1 pint) of water.[7,29] Saline is a useful agent in the care of mucositis, for irrigating a furred sore tongue,[30] and for use after brushing the teeth as an effective mouth rinse.

Sodium bicarbonate

This is an inexpensive, widely available, alkaline cleansing agent that is effective in dissolving tenacious mucus or a 'sloughy' mouth.[10,31] It can also be useful for a sensitive, dry mouth.[7,31] The recommended dilution is one teaspoonful in a pint of water.[32] However, it must be diluted correctly as otherwise it may cause superficial burns.[6] The taste of sodium bicarbonate is also unpleasant.

Chlorhexidine 0.2% (Corsydyl)

This is recommended as an effective cleansing agent in the prevention of plaque formation, and it is also effective against Gram-positive and Gram-negative infections, yeast and fungi.[7] It can cause reversible staining of the teeth. If it causes stinging or burning, dilute it 50:50 with water.[20] It should be used twice daily after meals and toothbrushing.[14] It is also available in a gel that can be applied directly to the teeth and gums.

Lemon and glycerine swabs

These are not recommended, although they have been used as moistening agents. However, they display no mechanical or chemical cleaning properties. The lemon increases salivation and glycerine absorbs water, so they actually increase dryness.[7,14]

Glycerine of thymol mouthwash

This is widely used and has a pleasant taste, but does little more than act as a rinse and a mouth-refresher.

Denture care

Denture care is an extremely important aspect of care of the patient's mouth, and can be associated with many oral problems.[33] For example, denture stomatitis is an inflammatory condition of the mucosa, which is manifested as erythema of the tissues supporting the denture, and can cause pain and discomfort. *Candida albicans* is associated with most cases of denture stomatitis.[33]

Denture do's and dont's!

Do's

- Do take dentures out at night.
- Do scrub dentures with soap or toothpaste and water.
- Do store them in fresh, changed daily cold Milton solution (hot Milton solution may cause denture bleaching to occur).
- Do remove, brush and clean after meals.[8]
- Do treat dentures with antifungal agents if the mouth is infected with *Candida* species.[33]
- Do check that the dentures are not rubbing or causing mucosal trauma. They may need altering or replacing altogether.
- Do consult with a local dentist for advice.

Don'ts

- Don't wear dentures if the mouth is sore or infected.
- Don't soak metal dentures or those with a metal frame in Milton solution (which may cause corrosion), but instead use chlorhexidine 0.2% (Corsydyl).[33]

Common oral complaints

All of these complaints require vigilant, thorough care by the health professional. Regular oral assessment and care must be ensured. Dental and medical opinions should be sought and a team approach adopted.

Adequate explanation to the patient and their family of the cause of their complaint may relieve anxiety.[34]

Xerostomia (dry mouth)

Xerostomia is particularly common in palliative care patients, and the degree of distress it causes *should not be underestimated*. Specific causes include radiotherapy to the head and neck, dehydration, depression, anxiety and oral infection. Drugs can also induce xerostomia (see Box 4.5 for a list). It is essential to check which drugs the patient is taking, and to find out whether they can be altered.

Box 4.5:   Drugs that cause xerostomia[35]

Anticholinergics
Anticonvulsants
Antidepressants
Antihistamines
Antihypertensives
Antineoplastics
Antipsychotics
Diuretics
Narcotic analgesics
Sympathomimetics

Symptoms of xerostomia include a red, smooth tongue, the corners of the mouth may become fissured, causing difficulty in swallowing and speech, and there is alteration to taste and difficulty in mastication (chewing).

Treatment

It is important to ensure that vigilant mouthcare is encouraged and sugary foods are avoided, as a dry mouth will lose the normal protective functions of saliva, and the teeth may consequently be more likely to decay. A dry mouth is also more likely to develop oral thrush.[37]

The following may be useful measures, as appropriate:

- pilocarpine – this drug is a muscarinic agonist and may be useful;[34,36]
- sodium bicarbonate mouthwashes;[37]
- artificial salivas (e.g. Saliva Orthana or Glandosane sprays);[34]
- jugs of iced water;
- sucking pieces of crushed ice;
- chilled jellies;
- encouraging an increase in fluid intake;[10]
- chilled wafers of pineapple to suck (provided that the mouth is not sore);[10,38,39]
- chewing sugar-free gum (e.g. En-de-kay);
- sugar-free sweets;
- rinsing a teaspoonful of salad oil round the mouth before going to bed;
- hand-held atomiser spray of water (available from chemists);
- the lips can be coated with paraffin jelly,[3,24] but should be cleaned first with normal saline;[3]
- alter the diet to suit dry mouth, by including more foods with a high moisture content (consult a dietitian as necessary);
- drink fluids with meals to facilitate mastication and sense of taste.

Oral thrush

Candidiasis is by far the commonest fungal infection seen in patients,[9] and is manifested as a white-yellowish plaque that can easily be removed, leaving a bleeding, painful surface.[3,9] However, it can also present as red, smooth mucosa, smooth tongue and angular cheilitis.[40]

Treatment

Conventional therapy consists of use of a nystatin suspension.[3,39] Dentures should also be treated with nystatin and toothbrushes should be replaced after any infection.[34] Nystatin diluted with water and then frozen into ice lollies is also soothing and provides an effective means of giving local relief.[9] Fluconazole is also recommended. A larger dose of fluconazole given as a single dose is especially useful if the patient has a very short time to live.[32] Oral care at this time should be performed regularly, frequently and thoroughly.

Painful mouth

Systemic analgesia may be required to treat oral pain, including the use of opioids.[39] Pain in the mouth, commonly due to mouth ulcers, can be greatly helped by benzydamine (Difflam) 0.15% as an oral rinse or gargle.[34] This can also be given in a spray form.[41]

Mouth ulcers can be treated with Orabase cream,[14,31,34] which forms a protective coat over mucosal surfaces and relieves painful ulcers on the tongue, gums and mucous membranes. Sucralfate, an anti-ulcer drug, can help to ease a painful, ulcerated mouth by binding to ulcerated tissue, creating a protective coating.[41] Choline salicylate gel (Bonjela) is also effective for mouth ulcers, but can cause stinging and pain on application.[39]

If chronic ulceration persists, or if the patient has a local tumour, an anaerobic antibiotic such as metronidazole syrup can be useful.[9,42] The use of a lignocaine gel is also recommended.

Furred tongue

A coated discoloured tongue results from the accumulation of dead epithelial cells, dried mucus and saliva on the tongue. Fungal infection may also be superimposed. The tongue may be white or grey, and can be black as a result of an overgrowth of pigment-producing bacteria, which is common in patients undergoing antibiotic treatment.[31]

As with all conditions of the mouth, extra vigilance should be maintained. The tongue can be gently brushed with a soft child's toothbrush (checking for soreness), or irrigated with saline, chlorhexidine 0.2% or sodium bicarbonate.[23,31] Pineapple chunks are also recommended,[34,39] as they contain the proteolytic enzyme ananase, which also cleans the mouth. Unsweetened tinned pineapple is preferable, although care should be taken if the mouth is sore. Another anecdotal recommendation is cider and soda water to help lift a thick coating from the tongue.[9] Effervescent vitamin C tablets dissolved on the tongue have also been suggested to be useful as a cleansing agent.[3,9]

Conclusion

Oral discomfort and pain have been identified as distressing symptoms which are often inadequately dealt with by the healthcare professional.[30] Ensuring that the patient has a clean healthy mouth is an essential part of nursing care. It is the responsibility of every professional to prioritise, and to aim to achieve good oral hygiene.

For the long-term patient for whom cure is no longer expected, especially a patient who has already lost so much (work, hobbies and mobility), to be able to converse freely, to smile, to laugh, and to taste and enjoy their food is of vital importance. This is the real essence of maintaining some quality of life.

Oral assessments are central to providing good oral care and, if possible, should involve both the patient and their family. Tools and agents for care must be employed carefully. Frequency and regularity of care may well be one of the most important factors in oral health. Above all, the mouth should *never* be neglected, and must be regarded as of equal importance to other areas that perhaps have a higher profile.

References

1   Kirkham S (1995) Sore mouth in context. *Eur J Palliative Care Suppl.* **2**: 3.

2   Holmes S (1996) Nursing management of oral care in older patients. *Nursing Times.* **92**: 37–9.

3   Krishnasamy H (1995) Oral problems in advanced cancer. *Eur J Cancer.* **4**: 173–7.

4   Jobbins J, Bagg J, Finlay IG *et al.* (1992) Oral and dental disease in terminally ill patients. *BMJ*, **304**: 1612.

5   Aldred MJ, Addy M, Bagg J *et al.* (1991) Oral health in the terminally ill – a cross-sectional pilot survey. *Specialist Care Dentistry.* **11**: 59–62.

6   Howarth H (1997) Mouthcare procedures for the very ill. *Nursing Times.* **83**: 25–7.

7   Madeya M (1996) Oral complications from cancer therapy. Part 2. Nursing implications for assessment and treatment. *Oncol Nurses Forum.* **23**: 808–18.

8   Gooch J (1985) Mouthcare. *Prof Nurse*. **Dec**: 77–8.

9   Ventafridda V *et al* (1993) Mouthcare. In: D Doyle, G Hanks and N MacDonald (eds) *Oxford Textbook of Palliative Medicine*. Oxford Medical Publications, Oxford.

10   Heals D (1993) A key to wellbeing. Oral hygiene in patients with advanced cancer. *Prof Nurse*. **Mar**: 391–8.

11   Holmes S (1991) The oral complications of specific anti-cancer therapy. *Int J Nurs Studies*. **28**: 343–60.

12   Turner G (1996) Oral care. *Nurs Standard*. **10**: 51–4.

13   Crosby C (1989) Method in mouthcare. *Nursing Times*. **85**: 38–41.

14   Davis R (1998) Mouthcare in oral cancer treatment – a nursing protocol. *Macmillan Nurse Suppl. 7*. **Jun**: 1–7.

15   Parker H (1994) Mouthcare in cancer. *Nursing Times*. **90**: 27–9.

16   Scully C (1995) Other causes of oral soreness. *Eur J Palliative Care Suppl*. **4**: 13–15

17   Holmes S (1996) Nursing management of oral care in older patients. *Nursing Times*. **92**: 37–9.

18   Hatton-Smith CK (1994) A last bastion of ritualised practice? A review of nurses' knowledge of oral healthcare. *Prof Nurse*. **Feb**: 304–8.

19   Eilers J, Berger AM and Petersen M (1988) Development, testing and application of the oral assessment guide. *Oncol Nurses Forum*. **15**: 325–30.

20   Feber T (1995) Mouthcare for patients receiving oral irradiation. *Prof Nurse*. **10**: 666–70.

21   Van Drimmelen J and Rollins HF (1969) Evaluation of a commonly used oral hygiene agent. *Nursing Res*. **18 (Jul/Aug)**: 327–32.

22   Roth PT and Creason NS (1986) Nurse administered oral hygiene – is there a scientific basis? *J Adv Nursing*. **11**: 323–31.

23   Jenkins D (1989) Oral care in the ICU. An important nursing role. *Nursing Standard*. **4**: 24–8.

24   Eldridge AD (1993) Mouthcare technique promotes patient comfort. *Oncol Nurse Forum*. **20**: 700.

25   Harris MD (1980) Tools for mouthcare. *Nursing Times*. **Feb 21**: 340–2.

26   Burglass EA (1995) Oral hygiene. *Br J Nursing*. **4**: 516–19.

27   Pearson LS (1996) A comparison of the ability of foam swabs and toothbrushes to remove dental plaque. Implications for nursing practice. *J Adv Nursing*. **23**: 62–9

28   Daeffler R (1980) Oral hygiene measures for patients with cancer. Part 1. *Cancer Nursing*. **3**: 347–55.

29   Maurer J (1977) Providing optimal oral health. *Nurs Clin North Am*. **12**: 671–85.

30 Shephard J, Page C, Sammon P *et al.* (1987) The mouth trap. *Nursing Times.* **83**: 25–7.

31 Hallett N (1984) Mouthcare. *Nursing Mirror.* **159**: 31–3.

32 Regnard C (1994) Single-dose fluconazole versus five-day ketoconazole in oral candidosis. *Palliative Med.* **8**: 72–3.

33 Walls A (1995) Dental causes of sore mouth. *Eur J Palliative Care Suppl.* **2**: 10–12.

34 Finegan W (1999) *HELP (Helpful Essential Links to Palliative Care)* (3e). Macmillan Cancer Relief/Centre for Macmillan Education, University of Dundee, Dundee.

35 Barnett J (1991) A reassessment of oral healthcare. *Prof Nurse.* **Sep**: 703–8.

36 Davies AN (1997) The management of xerostomia: a review. *Eur J Cancer Care.* **6**: 209–14.

37 Manson P (1999) A cure for a dry mouth. *Clin Management.* **Feb**: 28.

38 Krishnasamy M (1995) The nurse's role in oral care. *Eur J Palliative Care Suppl.* **2**: 8–9.

39 Regnard C and Tempest S (1998) Oral problems. In: C Regnard and S Tempest (eds) *A Guide to Symptom Relief in Advanced Disease.* Hochland and Hochland, Manchester.

40 Finlay I (1995) Oral fungal infections. *Eur J Palliative Care Suppl.* **2**: 4–7.

41 Soloman MA (1986) Oral sucralfate suspension for mucositis. *NEJM.* **315**: 459–60.

42 Macmillan Centre (1995) *The Patient has Mouth Problems and Bad Breath.* Spotlight 2.6, Spotlights 1–4 Series. Macmillan Center for Education, University of Dundee, Dundee.

To learn more

Regnard CFB and Tempest S (1998) *A Guide to Symptom Relief in Advanced Disease* (4e). Hochland and Hochland, Manchester.

Richardson A (1992) *Manual of Core Care Plans for Cancer Nursing* (1e). The Royal Marsden Hospital, Scutari Press and Royal College of Nursing, London.

Ventafridda V *et al.* (1993) Mouthcare. In: D Doyle, G Hanks and N Macdonald (eds) *Oxford Textbook of Palliative Care.* Oxford Medical Publications, Oxford.

Chapter 4: Answers to pre-reading exercise

1 Dry mouth.
2 Chemotherapy, radiotherapy, anxiety, depression and malnutrition.
3 Oral thrush, mouth ulcers and dry mouth.
4 Pen torch, tongue depressor, gloves and, if possible, a dental mirror.
5 Talking, taste, kissing, eating.

Lymphoedema

Mary Woods

Pre-reading exercise

Before reading this chapter, consider the following questions.

- What information might you need when assessing a patient with lymphoedema?
- What would you consider to be the primary goals of your intervention?
- What impact is lymphoedema likely to have on the patient and their family?

Introduction

There are many reasons why swelling (oedema) can appear in a limb, and the patient with advanced cancer in the palliative care setting requires a careful assessment of the cause of their swelling in order to establish the priorities in its management.

Oedema develops when, for a significant period of time, the volume of fluid entering the interstitial compartment of the tissues is greater than the rate at which the lymphatics can drain it. This may occur:

- if the capillary filtration rate is raised;
- if the transport capacity of the lymphatic system is reduced.

Raised capillary filtration rate

The capillary filtration rate may be raised, and therefore lead to swelling, without cancer necessarily being present. Continuous dependency of the legs – where the legs are below heart level in an elderly, immobile patient – will lead to swelling due to increased capillary pressure related to increased venous pressure. Similarly, venous insufficiency or obstruction can lead to swelling and subsequent leg ulceration.

In the patient with cancer, the capillary filtration rate will be raised if there is a lowered plasma protein concentration. The legs may become grossly swollen, and this type of oedema frequently indicates the advanced stages of disease.

Reduced lymphatic system transport capacity

The transport capacity of the lymphatic system is reduced if damage or obstruction have occurred. This has the effect of reducing the available drainage routes, and swelling can result.

The lymphatic system may be damaged following cancer-related treatment involving lymph-node areas. Surgery and radiotherapy to lymph-node areas of the axilla and groin are examples of cases where this may happen. The swelling may develop at any time following the initial cancer treatment.[2]

Obstruction of the lymphatic system can also occur when there is tumour growth in lymph-node areas. The lymph flow may then become severely restricted and swelling develops.

Assessment

The goal of palliative care is to achieve the best possible quality of life for the patient. Thus it involves promoting physical and psychological comfort within the limitations imposed by a disease that has become life-threatening. If swelling is present, the patient's needs and aims must always be considered, and their choices and priorities respected. A careful assessment of the patient will aid the development of a realistic and appropriate management plan. The burden of treatment should not exceed the benefit to be gained, and it is therefore important to ascertain the patient's views concerning the most appropriate means of managing the swelling, to ensure that they are not overburdened with difficult and unrealistic daily regimes. Box 5.1 outlines the different aspects of the assessment process that can be used.

Box 5.1:   Assessment

General information: to establish the cause and type of swelling.
Physical examination: to assess the extent of the swelling.
Psychological and psychosocial assessment: to establish the influence of the swelling.

General information

Establishing the cause and type of swelling is the first step in the assessment process. In advanced cancer, there are often a number of factors that may contribute to the appearance of swelling, and by obtaining some general information from the patient, or their medical history, an understanding can be gained of why the swelling has developed. The patient's past and current medical history will help to distinguish between swelling due to obstructive causes and that due to other more central causes. Fluid-retaining drugs may exacerbate swelling, and knowledge of any allergies should be recorded. It is helpful to find out how long the swelling has been present and whether it has changed in any way.

Physical examination

In order to establish the extent of the swelling, a physical examination of the swollen and surrounding area is necessary. The visual appearance of the limb can provide information about the condition and integrity of the skin and the presence of any infection or complicating factors that may influence management of the swelling. Repeated episodes of infection in a swollen limb can impair lymph drainage and thus exacerbate the swelling even further. The function, movement and sensations or pain that are experienced in the swollen limb can also be established during this stage of the assessment, in order to determine whether involvement of other members of the multidisciplinary team in the patient's care should be considered. The skills of a physiotherapist and an occupational therapist can be invaluable in maximising the patient's potential with regard to limb movement and function when swelling is present.

Psychological and psychosocial assessment

The patient with advanced cancer may have a number of problems of which the swelling may be only one, and of less importance than the others. By establishing the influence of the swelling on the patient's individual circumstances, their psychological and psychosocial needs can be considered. Even when the patient's life expectancy is of the order of months or years, their hobbies, interests, occupation and self-image may still be important to them. Management of the swelling will therefore be more intensive than when the patient is in the last few days or weeks of life. By establishing a rapport with the patient and their family or friends, the influence that the swelling may have on the patient can be considered.[3]

A thorough assessment process will enable the likely outcomes to be established and an *appropriate*, *realistic* and *individualised* treatment plan to be developed which can have a dramatic impact on the patient's quality of life.

Management of swelling

The approach to the management of swelling in a patient with advanced cancer can be considered within the framework outlined in Box 5.2. However, it is important to take into consideration the factors established during the assessment, together with the patient's wishes.

Box 5.2:   Management of swelling

Reduction.
Control.
Palliation.

Education, advice and information concerning the nature of the swelling should be offered to the patient, and realistic outcomes of the treatment must be explained. A combination of treatments may be used, depending on the type of swelling and its severity. The treatments that may be offered are illustrated in Box 5.3.

Box 5.3:   Elements of treatment

Skin care: to promote skin integrity.
Exercise: to maintaim limb function.
Massage: to stimulate lymph drainage.
External support: to promote lymph drainage.

Reduction of the swelling

This approach to management of the swelling may be chosen if the main aim is to enhance the drainage of the congested lymphatic routes, and to reduce and then control the swelling.

Management will include appropriate skin care as illustrated in Box 5.4, in order to promote the integrity of the skin. Movement and exercise are promoted in order to maintain limb and joint mobility and function. External support to the swollen limb may be provided with a course of multi-layer compression bandages or compression hosiery.

Box 5.4:   Skin care to promote skin integrity

Daily skin hygiene.
Daily skin moisturising with a bland unperfumed moisturising cream.
Antiseptic treatment of all breaks, cuts or abrasions to the skin.

Lymphatic drainage can be stimulated with the use of simple self-massage or manual lymphatic drainage, both of which are outlined in Box 5.5. Reduction should always be followed by control of the swelling.

Box 5.5:   Manual lymphatic drainage and self-massage

Manual lymph drainage: a specialised form of skin massage using gentle, highly specialised hand movements performed by a fully trained manual lymph drainage therapist.
Self-administered massage: a simplified form of skin massage based on manual lymph drainage which can be taught by a lymphoedema therapist and be self-administered by the patient or their relative.

Control of the swelling

When reduction of the swelling has been achieved, or if it is an unrealistic aim because the patient is too ill or frail, or unable to tolerate the methods of treatment involved in reduction, control of the swelling can prevent a worsening of the situation and provide some comfort for the patient. This approach to management will include skin care and passive or active exercise of the swollen limb. In addition, external support may be provided by bandages adapted to suit the patient's needs, or compression garments which will control the swelling and relieve some of the tension and tightness that may be felt in the limb.

Palliation of the symptoms

The emphasis on treatment is:

● to reduce any discomfort experienced; and
● to optimise the quality of the patient's remaining life.

Symptoms may include the following:

● pain;
● heaviness;
● bursting in the tissues of the swollen limb;
● aching in the joints or muscles.

The approach to management of the symptoms will be individually tailored, with the main focus being on comfort. Skin care and passive exercise of the swollen limb may be used, and some relief of tension and tightness in the tissues can sometimes be achieved by the use of gentle external support.

Complications

Patients with advanced cancer who develop swelling may experience a variety of problems relating to the swelling, some of which are more complex and difficult to address than others. A multidisciplinary approach with appropriate management strategies provides the opportunity for optimum care and support for the patient when these potentially distressing complications develop.

Skin problems

The maintenance of skin integrity, in order to minimise the risks of infection, is a major factor in the management of swelling and the relief of symptoms associated with the latter. The main components of skin care are illustrated in Box 5.4.

In advanced cancer, weeping and ulceration of the affected limb can occur, and fungating lesions may develop within the swollen area. Although these problems can be difficult to deal with, choice of the correct non-adherent dressing (e.g. Alleveyn, Sorbsan) secured with a light retention bandage (thus avoiding the use of dressing tape) will promote patient comfort without compromising the fragile condition of the skin.

Large quantities of fluid may leak from the swollen area if lymphorrhoea develops. This frequently follows a small cut or break in the skin due to trauma, and presents a real risk of infection. The fluid loss cannot be controlled by the use of simple dressings alone, and a recent survey among palliative care units found the use of gentle pressure provided by compression bandages to be the most widely employed method of managing lymphorrhoea.[4]

Truncal swelling

One of the most distressing problems that patients with swelling may encounter is when swelling extends beyond the root of a limb to involve the genital, vulval or chest wall area. Movement of fluid is frequently limited by the obstruction of tumour, but some relief may be achieved by the use of self-massage or by manual lymphatic drainage therapy provided by a skilled practitioner.

Function

The movement and function of a swollen limb can be impeded by tumour pressing on nerves, and leading to a variety and differing degree of symptoms in the limb. These may range from tingling and numbness to complete loss of sensation and movement.

Brachial plexus neuropathy is often progressive and accompanied by pain, requiring the skills of the multidisciplinary team to relieve discomfort and maximise function within the limitations imposed by the condition.

Summary

Lymphoedema is a chronic condition which is unlikely to resolve completely, particularly if the sufferer has advanced cancer. It is a unique and individual experience for each patient which can affect them in a wide variety of ways and differing degrees. The skills of the therapist are needed to establish the main priorities in the patient's care in order to achieve the best quality of life for them within the limitations imposed on them by the swelling.

Chapter 5:   Questions

1 Name two reasons why oedema may develop.
2 List the three areas of the assessment process that can be used when a patient has swelling.
3 Name the approach to the management of swelling that may be used when reduction of the swelling either has been achieved or is an unrealistic aim.
4 List the four elements of treatment that can be used to manage lymphoedema.
5 Name one complication that may be observed in the patient with swelling.

References

1   Levick JR (1991) *An Introduction to Cardiovascular Physiology*. Butterworths, London.

2   Logan V (1995) Incidence and prevalence of lymphoedema: a literature review. *J Clin Nursing*. 4: 213–19.

3   Woods M (1995) Sociological factors and psychological implications of lymphoedema. *Int J Palliative Nursing*. 1. 17–20.

4   Ling J, Duncan A, Laverty D and Hardy J (1997) Lymphorrhoea in palliative care. *Eur J Palliative Care*. 4: 50–2.

To learn more

British Lymphology Society (1997) *Definitions Relating to the Population and Needs of People with or at Risk of Developing Chronic Oedema*. British Lymphology Society, Caterham. Surrey.

Macmillan Cancer Relief (1997) *Macmillan Lymphoedema Pilot Project*. Macmillan Cancer Relief, London.

Chapters 5:   Answers

1 Raised capillary filtration rate, and reduced transport capacity of the lymphatic system.
2 General information, physical examination and psychological and psychosocial assessment.
3 Control of the swelling.
4 Skin care, exercise, massage and external support.
5 Truncal problems, skin problems or functional problems.

CHAPTER 6

Wound care

Mark Collier

Pre-reading exercise

Reflect upon a patient whom you recently cared for who had a malignant fungating lesion. Write down brief notes relating to the specific wound management interventions that you either undertook or observed another healthcare professional undertake on the patient's behalf. Ask a colleague to do the same, and then discuss and compare each other's notes. When you have read this chapter, return to your notes, highlighting any changes that you might make to your approach should you have the opportunity to nurse a similar patient in the future. Discuss your thoughts with your colleague, identifying the rationale that underpins any changes you may have highlighted.

Introduction

The aim of this chapter is to introduce the reader to several of the many aspects of wound care that are relevant to and important for the overall holistic management of patients with malignant (fungating) lesions.

At the end of this chapter, the reader should be able to:

- discuss the epidemiology and pathophysiology of fungating wounds;
- have a better understanding of how to recognise such wounds;
- understand the relevance of an holistic patient assessment in order to plan appropriate care interventions;
- be able to discuss specific aspects of wound management relevant to the patient with a fungating lesion;
- discuss a number of wound management materials (dressings) which might be utilised for relevant patient care and identify the rationale for their choice.

'Fungating wounds are visible markers of an underlying disease.'[1]

The term 'fungating wounds' refers to the infiltration into and proliferation of malignant cells through the epidermis of the skin, the origin of which may be a local tumour or a distant primary lesion due to metastatic activity.[2] These tumours may grow rapidly, and if so they often take on a cauliflower-like appearance. However, they may also ulcerate and form shallow craters that can be complicated by the presence of an associated sinus or fistula.[3] Because of the amount of wound exudate that is normally associated with them, the latter group are also commonly described as 'malodorous' wounds.

A malodorous wound may be defined as 'any wound assessed as being offensive (smelly) by either the patient, the practitioner or both'.[1] Nevertheless it is important to remember that a variety of wound aetiologies (e.g. pressure ulcers, leg ulcers, traumatic wounds) can be malodorous without being malignant, whereas in the majority of cases fungating wounds will have an associated odour at some point during their treatment.[4]

Epidemiology

Epidemiological studies of this subject within the UK, are unfortunately rare, with most reported data being based on estimations.[5] Thomas, following his retrospective survey utilising information collected mainly from radiotherapy and oncology units, discussed the most reliable data.[6] Respondents were asked to record how many fungating wounds they had seen over the previous 4 weeks, and to indicate whether the resultant figure was typical of an average month. They were also asked to estimate how many cases of this particular wound type they had encountered during the previous year. From the 114 replies, a monthly total of 295 fungating wounds was reported, with an annual total of 2417 such wounds. In addition, Thomas reported the location of fungating wounds as follows: breast, 62%; head and face, 24%; groin and genitals, 3%; back, 3%; others, 8%.

Pathophysiology

Tumour infiltration of the skin involves the spread of malignant cells along pathways that offer minimal resistance, such as tissue planes, blood and lymph capillaries and the perineural spaces.[7]

Abnormalities in the vascularisation of both the lesion and the surrounding tissues are often associated with tumour formation, although the mechanisms involved in the control of this process are not yet fully understood. However, hypoxic regions within the margins of the tumour will occur as a result of fluctuations in the blood supply and therefore cell perfusion. Deficiencies may also arise in the lymphatic system, affecting interstitial tissue drainage when interstitial fluid pressures exceed extravascular pressures and lead to the collapse of vessel walls. The haemostasis of the blood, lymph, interstitial and cellular environments may therefore be severely disturbed by this process.[3] For example, rapid proliferation of tumour cells may occur in the acidic pH conditions of extracellular fluid, which in turn will affect the tension within the blood cells.[8]

Tissue hypoxia itself in a fungating wound can be a significant problem, as anaerobic organisms flourish in accessible necrotic tissue – a characteristic of the majority of fungating tumours. The malodorous volatile fatty acids that are released as a metabolic end-product are responsible for the characteristic smell and profuse exudate often associated with these wound types, the exudate being attributed to the activity of bacterial enzymes (proteases) and their role in tissue breakdown. Stagnant exudate may also be responsible for any odour in the wound,[1,9] and therefore needs to be considered carefully and incorporated into wound assessment criteria by all practitioners.

Recognition of the problem

Patients with fungating wounds may present at an early age with advanced conditions, or only when metastatic disease is evident. This may be recognised by the patient because of the development of unanticipated additional lesions. Another author has previously attempted to identify some of the many complex reasons that cause some patients (especially women with breast lesions[10] and, in this author's experience, men with testicular lesions) to delay seeking diagnosis and treatment of their 'suspect' growth.

Diagnosis is based on histological assessment, and cultures taken from the surface of these wounds usually confirm the presence of anaerobic organisms such as *Bacteroides*. If the presence of these organisms is not dealt with appropriately, the result will be the production of by-products such as propionic, lactic and succinic acids, which if not controlled by the use of appropriate absorbent dressing materials (e.g. alginates) will quickly result in maceration of and damage to the tissue surrounding the original lesion. Maceration may be defined as the stripping/excoriation of the epidermis due to the 'prolonged' presence of toxins on the skin.

Identification of these metabolic end-products usually involves gas–liquid chromatography analysis. This technique is a practical, inexpensive procedure that can be undertaken in the clinical laboratory.

It should be emphasised that the presence of a fungating wound is not necessarily an intractable problem, and therefore the medical aims of treatment and patient management may be identified in the first instance as follows:

- control of growth of the tumour;
- arresting surface haemorrhage;
- if at all possible, preserving or restoring the viability of the patient's tissues.

Treatment protocols may therefore include one or more of the following:

- radiotherapy;
- surgery;
- laser therapy;
- cytotoxic or hormone replacement therapy;
- control of any symptomatology displayed by the patient either during or after these treatments.

The effects of the above need to be assessed as part of the holistic patient assessment, addressed sympathetically and all observations utilised in order to direct appropriate interventions, including those local to the wound (i.e. the use of wound management materials).

Patient assessment – a holistic perspective

It is imperative that all practitioners involved in the care of these patients adopt an holistic approach to the management of both the patient and their wound – acknowledging the interrelationship between the two – in order to facilitate both objective and quality-management strategies.

It could be argued that the use of a nursing model, such as the Roper, Logan and Tierney Activities of Living Model,[11] can aid the identification of the patient's problems and needs, and may also be used by all members of the multidisciplinary team in order to plan, structure and implement interventions designed to have a positive impact on the patient's current and future lifestyle.

Maintaining a safe environment

This is important in order to reduce the risk of infection (either local or systemic), as this may complicate both wound assessment and the overall patient wound management plan. Wound infection can be the cause of further discomfort for the patient, and may result in odours being associated with the lesion as a result of anaerobic activity,[1] as for example with bacteroidal colonisation.

Nearly 100% of all wounds (particularly chronic wounds that have accessible necrotic tissue within their margins) will be colonised by some organism, most commonly the host's *Staphylococcus aureus*. However, the presence of bacteria or slough within the wound margins alone may not be of any clinical significance.[12] An infected wound may be defined as one that has been colonised by organisms that have become pathogenic and resulted in an adverse host reaction (e.g. pus production or additional tissue breakdown).

Communication with the patient

This is crucial to their psychological well-being. It is important to keep the patient informed of their general condition, prognosis (especially if they seek clarification of this), and in particular the state of their wound, as anxiety caused by a lack of information can impair and adversely affect the patient's natural healing potential.[13]

Occasionally the malignant lesion may invade the patient's head and neck region.[14] If this happens the patient's speech may be adversely affected and it may therefore be appropriate to encourage them to write down all that they would otherwise have spoken.[15]

Breathing

This ensures adequate ventilation and helps to maintain an oxygen-rich supply to the wound, thereby optimising any healing potential. Both progressive disease and the ageing process can alter this process. The specific evidence for the role of oxygen in wound healing, which can often appear contradictory, has been discussed elsewhere.[16]

Eating and drinking

A balanced intake is important to ensure the provision of essential nutrients such as protein, vitamins (A, B_{12} and C), minerals (zinc and iron) and carbohydrates. If it is not practicable for the patient to take oral supplements because of the side-effects of any chosen 'treatment' modality, then the nutrition and dietetics department should be informed if in the hospital setting, or else the community dietitian should be contacted and advice sought about an alternative approach to the delivery of the nutrients as appropriate.

Elimination

This should be as normal as possible. Urinary or faecal incontinence may be either a concern or an actual problem for the patient if the malignant lesion is in the perianal region, or is the cause of a fistula involving either the bladder or the bowel. In many cases suprapubic urinary catheters will be inserted and colostomies performed electively in order to alleviate the patient's symptomatology.[17]

Maintaining body temperature

Hypothermia has previously been reported to delay the healing process significantly,[18] and therefore any interventions such as the use of cold solutions or leaving the wound exposed for prolonged periods of time (e.g. when another colleague is expected to visit the 'clinical area' in order to assess it or give an opinion on the ongoing management of the wound) should be avoided. Pyrexia may be an indication of wound infection. It has previously been reported that if an infection is inappropriately treated and the pyrexia is prolonged, for each degree rise in body temperature the metabolic demands of the patient are increased by 10%.[19]

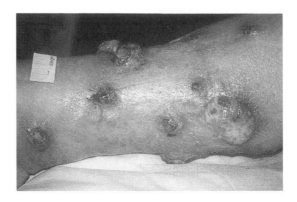

Figure 6.1   The lower limb of a patient with malignant melanoma, with multiple lesions evident.

Mobilisation

If the mobility of either an individual limb or the whole body is reduced this can result in associated joint stiffness and muscle atrophy and induce circulatory stasis, which may predispose the patient to the development of pressure ulcers[20] or deep vein thrombosis, further complicating the management of their medical condition.

Expressing sexuality

Disfiguring lesions (*see* Figure 6.1) can increase the patient's anxiety and sense of isolation because of an altered body image.[21] Often feelings that the patient experiences range from embarrassment ('nobody will want to talk to me') through to depression, and may be the sole reason for a change in the patient's lifestyle. James Partridge, Director of Changing Faces and himself a patient who has experienced a facially disfiguring wound) has identified a typical set of reactions and feelings that this group of patients may encounter, which he has summarised as the SCARED syndrome.[22]

	You		*They*	
Feel	*Behave*		*Behave*	*Feel*
Self-conscious	Submissive	S	Staring	Sympathy
Conspicuous	Clumsy	C	Curious	Caution
Angry	Apathetic	A	Awkward	Anguish
Resentful	Regressive	R	Rude	Reluctance
Empty	Excluded	E	Evasive	Embarrassment
Different	Defenceless	D	Distance	Dread

Psychological issues

When for whatever reason the patient's anxiety level is increased, it has been reported that their perception of pain – related to any wound management techniques – can also be significantly heightened.[23] In addition, any pain experienced in association with fungating wounds may be increased by the fear of visualising the lesion and further exacerbated by odour or the fear of dying.[24]

The main source of malodour related to skin ulcers such as fungating wounds (other than stagnant exudate) has been reported to be two key impact odours which can trigger a gagging or vomit reflex in patients and carers alike. There is evidence that this particular malodour is detectable and persistent, thereby increasing the patient's self-consciousness about it, which may inhibit them from inviting friends to visit.[25]

Dying

The ideal aim of wound healing may be unrealistic in the terminally ill patient, and the choice of dressing materials used may therefore be influenced more by the need to maintain or enhance the patient's quality of life.[26] Nevertheless, it is essential to consider the patient's choice of care setting at an early stage, especially if the tumour is malignant and the prognosis poor. Should it be the hospital, at home or in a hospice? Every effort must be made to ensure that the patient achieves as peaceful a death as possible with all relevant support and services available at the time.[27]

Sleeping

This is an essential factor in tissue regeneration, as it encourages the release of testosterone, prolactin, somatotrophin and growth hormone.[28] The patient should be encouraged to rest as much as possible, especially if they are receiving aggressive rather than palliative therapies. Occasionally, mild sedatives and relaxants may be prescribed to facilitate periods 'at rest'.

Diversional therapy

Patients with fungating wounds at all stages of treatment should be encouraged to adopt as normal a lifestyle as possible, continuing to pursue any hobbies and maintain interests such as photography, listening to music, watching television or even gentle gardening.

Religion

This is very important to many patients, and therefore every effort should be made, whatever the care setting, to meet the identified needs of the individual.

Principles of wound assessment

Although the principles of wound assessment have been discussed in detail previously by this author,[9] it is still important to consider the specifics of assessment (relevant to the patient with a fungating wound) in order to ensure that any planned interventions do not adversely interact with any course of treatment currently being undertaken, examples of which have previously been highlighted.

The process of wound assessment should incorporate the practitioner's knowledge of relevant anatomy and physiology (including the normal wound-healing process), collection of both objective and subjective data, analysis and interpretation of the information obtained, and identification of the patient's problems and needs through discussion, leading to subsequent goal-planning and care regimens.[29]

Specific wound assessment should highlight the characteristics and nature of the wound, such as its location, the size of the lesion, the percentage of devitalised material noted within the wound margins, the amount and nature of any exudate being produced by the wound, whether any odour can be associated with the lesion, the nature and type of pain that can be directly attributed to the fungating wound (and the effects of this on the patient's activities of daily living), and finally the current state of the surrounding skin immediately adjacent to the wound itself.[4]

Noting wound location can often aid identification of the cause of the wound, especially in the case of chronic wound types (the classification most relevant to fungating lesions). In addition, it can alert the practitioner to potential and actual problems that may be experienced by both the patient and the nurse in dealing with the lesion. In the patient's case, a fungating wound close to the axilla or any joint may impair normal movements undertaken by the patient, thus affecting their normal activities of daily living. For the nurse, the location may highlight difficulties in securing any chosen secondary dressing material without further adverse effects being experienced by the patient.

Measuring wound size is now generally regarded as important, as well as keeping accurate visual records of the change in surface area of an open wound in order to identify any trend associated with the latter. Is the wound showing signs of improvement? Is it deteriorating?

There are a number of methods available for assessing wounds visually, including computer mapping, polaroid-type photography (incorporating a scale such as a paper ruler within the frame near to the wound) and tracing wounds using a clean transparent film or sheet. However, in this author's experience it is not advisable to trace these wound types, as local bleeding from the surface of the wound may often be induced as a result of contact of the tracing material with very friable tissues.

Wound photography does provide a two-dimensional representation of the wound. However, there are difficulties in using the results for comparative purposes, and previous authors have highlighted the need to ensure that the camera angle, focal length and patient position are consistent.[30,31] In addition, but perhaps more importantly, the sensitive position of the wound may preclude the use of this data-collection method in the first instance – that is, until a positive rapport has been established between the practitioner and the patient.

An additional potential problem associated with the use of photography is that the full extent of the wound may not be seen, as in the case of undermining. In an attempt to combat this, ultrasound imaging has been considered as an assessment tool for fungating wounds.[32]

Grocott has previously discussed the equipment used and the nature of ultrasound imaging and its suitability as an assessment tool for this wound type, concluding that the method was rejected 'on the grounds that the intrusion to the patient was not justified relative to the quality of the information obtained'.[32]

Assessing the wound bed/percentage of devitalised tissue

The use of classification tools such as those identified previously by this author[9] is important in order to take into account the amount of tissue destruction noted within the wound margins and to assess the major characteristics of the tissues seen within those margins. Are they necrotic, sloughy or granulating?

Assessing wound odour and the skin surrounding the wound

It is difficult to assess the presence of odour objectively. Nevertheless, when a fungating wound is being assessed it is the subjective reporting by the patient of the presence of any odour, which should guide the subsequent treatment regimes. This is especially important as, as in the opinion of this author, nurses can become desensitised to odour as a result of repeated exposure to wounds with similar symptomatology.

The condition of the patient's skin surrounding the wound can indicate the presence of wound infection (the clinical signs of which include inflammation, localised erythema, heat or pain), and highlight a problem of tissue maceration caused by excessive production of exudate that is inappropriately allowed to remain on the patient's skin.

Assessing wound pain

This involves observing the depth of the wound as well as noting critical factors such as the type of pain reported by the patient, its severity, duration and any precipitating factors. For example, is pain only reported at night when the patient has time to focus on his or her body, as the number of distracters is usually reduced at this time?

Documentation of wound assessments

There is evidence that wound assessment can be enhanced by the use of a reliable and systematic chart such as those devised by Morison[33] and Flanagan.[34]

As a consequence of systematic wound assessment, it could be argued that practitioners should be able to answer the following four questions.

1 What is the aetiology and location of the wound?
2 How should the wound be graded using an 'objective' grading tool?
3 Based on the identified wound grading, what is the primary treatment objective for this wound as seen?
4 What treatment regime is required in order to facilitate the achievement of the identified treatment objective?

As has already been highlighted, the primary goal of wound healing may not be appropriate for all patients with fungating wounds. However, it could be argued that treatment objectives identified as a result of the assessment process should include the following.

- Optimise the patient's healing potential.
- Optimise the local healing environment.
- Reduce the effects of any complications associated with the lesion.
- Reduce any offensive odour(s).
- Reduce any associated wound pain.

Principles of wound management

Although the principles of optimum wound management should always be remembered,[16] in this author's opinion it is the problems as perceived by the patient that

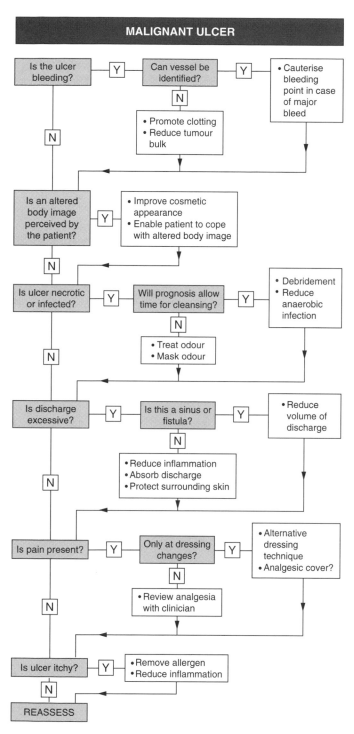

Figure 6.2 Management guidelines for a patient with a fungating wound (after Saunders and Regnard[35]).

should structure the overall wound management plan, in addition to those identified by practitioners.

Unless otherwise prescribed, the wound cleansing agent of choice – if indicated at all – would be normal saline 0.9%. In addition, topical antibacterial agents such as metronidazole gel (otherwise known as Metrotop) may be used in conjunction with appropriate dressing materials,[36] in order to aid the control of any perceived wound odours as discussed previously.

Wound management materials (dressings) to be considered

Grocott has previously identified the following principles which should be considered when choosing a wound dressing material as part of the overall management plan for a patient with fungating wounds:[37]

- the control of pain through the maintenance of optimum humidity at the wound site by using dressings that do not adhere to the tumour;
- facilitation of wound debridement with removal of excess exudate and toxic materials to prevent dehydration and control odour;
- topical antibiotics/antibacterial agents to control odour as appropriate;
- removal of dressings without trauma;
- restoration of body symmetry by the use of cavity dressings;
- achievement of cosmetic acceptability without the need for bulky secondary dressings;
- control of bleeding when it occurs by the use of haemostatic dressings such as alginates.

Bearing the above principles in mind, the following wound management and dressing protocol might be considered[27] (*see also* the Wound Management Protocol):

- activated charcoal – odorous lesions, but not if heavily exuding;
- alginates (flat/ribbon/packing) – exuding and/or bleeding wounds;
- hydrocolloid sheets – lightly exuding wounds, or for protection of the surrounding skin;
- semi-permeable film membranes – for protection only and then only if the surrounding skin is intact;
- foams/hydropolymers – for exuding wounds, and may occasionally be used in conjunction with alginates;
- secondary dressings of choice, remembering not to compromise the patient's skin by inappropriate use of dressing materials or adhesive tapes/fixations.

The primary functions of the above interactive wound management materials (dressing products identified by generic classification) have previously been discussed in detail by this author elsewhere.[16]

Conclusion

As with any wound management scenario, it is important for all practitioners to evaluate their interventions at intervals dictated by the systematic and holistic assessment of the patient and their wound, as discussed earlier in this chapter.

Caring for a patient with a fungating lesion can be both challenging and rewarding for practitioners, especially for the nurse who is ideally placed to enhance the quality of the care that the patient receives, either as a result of their own actions or by identifying the need for other members of the multidisciplinary team, further to their own holistic assessment of the patient under their care.

'Remember, if you keep in mind the patient's best interests you will be both their best friend and advocate as well as their carer.'[27]

Chapter 6:   Questions

Highlight or tick the correct answer for each of the following questions.

1 Which of the following has been reported to be the most common anatomical site for the development of a fungating wound?
a Abdomen
b Breast
c Chest
d Digits

2 In which of the following 'local' environments may rapid proliferation of tumour cells occur?
  a Moist acidic
  b Moist alkaline
  c Moist hypoxic
  d Dry anoxic.

3 For which of the following is an holistic approach to patient assessment crucial?
  a To confirm that the nurse knows best and has everything under control.
  b To ensure that the patient is able to look after him- or herself with minimal intervention from carers.
  c To plan, structure and implement care interventions which have a negative impact on the patient.
  d To plan, structure and implement care interventions which have a positive impact on the patient.

4 The principle on which modern wound management interventions are based involves ensuring that the following environment is maintained at the wound interface.
  a Warm and dry

b Cold and dry
c Warm and moist
d Cold and moist.

5 When attempting to measure the size of a fungating lesion, all of the following techniques may be considered except one. Which is it?
a Computer mapping
b Two-dimensional photography
c Wound mapping
d Ultrasound.

6 All of the following wound management materials have been identified as appropriate for the management of malignant fungating lesions except one. Which is it?
a Alginates
b Foams
c Hydrocolloids
d Particulates.

References

1   Neal K (1991) Treating fungating wounds *Nursing Times*. **87**: 85–6.

2   Mortimer P (1993) Skin problems in palliative care: medical aspects. In: D Doyle, G Hanks and N Macdonald (eds) *Oxford Textbook of Palliative Medicine*. Oxford Medical Publications, Oxford.

3   Collier M (1998) The assessment of patients with malignant fungating wounds – an holistic approach. Part one. *Nursing Times*. 93: Suppl.

4   Collier M (1997) The holistic management of fungating wounds. *Nursing Notes*. **14**: 2–5.

5   Ivetic O and Lyne P (1990) Fungating and ulcerating malignant lesions: a review of the literature. *J Adv Nursing*. **15**: 83–8.

6   Thomas S (1992) *Current Practices in the Management of Fungating Lesions and Radiation-Damaged Skin*. Surgical Materials Testing Laboratory, Bridgend.

7   Willis R (1973) *The Spread of Tumours in the Human Body* (3e). Butterworths, London.

8   Grocott P (1995) The palliative management of fungating malignant wounds. *J Wound Care*. **4**: 240–42.

9   Collier M (1994) Assessing a wound – RCN Nursing Update (Unit 29). *Nursing Standard*. **8 (Suppl.)**: 3–8.

10   Fairburn K (1993) Towards better care for women. Understanding fungating breast lesions. *Prof Nurse*. **8**: 204–12.

11   Roper N, Logan W and Tierney A (1985) *The Elements of Nursing*. Churchill Livingstone, Edinburgh.

12   Ayliffe G, Geddes A, Lowbury E and Williams J (1992) *Control of Hospital-acquired Infection* (3e). Chapman and Hall, London.

13   Boore J (1978) *Prescription for Recovery.* Royal College of Nursing, London.

14   McElney M (1993) The psychological effects of head and neck surgery. *J Wound Care.* **2:** 47–52.

15   Saunders S (1993) Mutual support. Wound Care Nursing Supplement. *Nursing Times.* **32:** 76–82.

16   Collier M (1996) Principles of optimum wound management. *Nursing Standard.* **10:** 47–52.

17   Carville K (1995) Caring for cancerous wounds in the community. *J Wound Care.* **4:**66–8.

18   Collier M (1990) Wound assessment – making informed choices. *Practice Nursing.* **Nov:** 17–18.

19   Moody M (1992) Problem wounds: a nursing challenge – RCN Nursing Update (Unit 17). *Nursing Standard.* **7**(6): 3–8.

20   Collier M (1989) *Pressure Sore Development and Prevention.* Educational Leaflet 3. Wound Care Society, Huntingdon.

21   Topping A (1992) The trauma of burns. *Wound Management.* **2:** 8–9.

22   Partridge J (1990) *Changing Faces – the Challenge of Facial Disfigurement.* Penguin, Harmondsworth.

23   Hargreaves A and Lander J (1989) Use of trancutaneous nerve stimulation for post-operative pain. *Nursing Res.* **38:** 159–61.

24   Hollingworth H (1997) *Pain.* Educational Leaflet 4. Wound Care Society, Huntingdon.

25   Van Toller S (1994) Invisible wounds: the effects of skin ulcer malodours. *J Wound Care.* **3:** 103–5.

26   Franks P (1998) Quality of life as an outcome indicator. In: M Morison, C Moffatt, S Bale and J Bridel-Nixon (eds) *Nursing Management of Chronic Wounds.* Mosby, London.

27   Collier M (1998) The assessment of patients with malignant fungating wounds – an holistic approach. Part two. *Nursing Times.* **93** (**Suppl.**): 1–4.

28   Torrance C (1990) Sleep and wound healing. *Surg Nurse.* **3:** 16–20.

29   Kratz C (1979) *The Nursing Process.* Ballière-Tindall, London.

30   Griffen J, Tolley E, Tooms R *et al.* (1993) A comparison of photographic and transparency based methods for measuring wound surface area. *Physical Therapy.* **73:** 117–22.

31   Thomas A and Wysocki A (1990) The healing wound: a comparison of three clinically useful methods of measurement. *Decubitus.* **3:** 18–25.

32   Grocott P (1995) Assessment of fungating wounds. *J Wound Care.* **4:** 333–6.

33   Morison M (1992) Wound care – a problem solving approach. RCN Nursing Update. *Nursing Standard*. **6 Suppl**: 37: 9–14.

34   Flanagan M (1998) *Wound Management*. ACE Series. Churchill Livingstone, Edinburgh.

35   Saunders J and Regnard C (1989) Management of malignant ulcers – a flow diagram. *Palliative Medicine*. **3**: 153–5.

36   Thomas S (1990) *Wound Management and Dressings*. Pharmaceutical Press, London.

37   Grocott P (1992) Application of the principles of modern wound management for complex wounds. In: *Proceedings of the First European Conference on the Advances of Wound Management*. EMAP, London.

To learn more

Kratz C (1979) *The Nursing Process*. Ballière-Tindall, London.

Orem D (1985) *Concepts of Practice* (3e). McGraw-Hill, St Louis.

Grocott P (1992) Application of the principles of modern wound management for complex wounds. In: *Proceedings of the First European Conference on the Advances of Wound Management*. EMAP, London.

Collier M (1996) Principles of optimum wound management. *Nursing Standard*. **10**: 47–52.

Saunders S (1993) Mutual support. Wound Care Nursing Supplement. *Nursing Times*. **32**: 76–82.

Chapter 6:   Answers

1 b
2 a
3 d
4 c
5 c
6 d

CHAPTER 7

Terminal restlessness

Jo Cooper

Pre-reading exercise

Think about a patient whom you have nursed recently where restlessness and agitation featured in the last days or hours of life. Answer the following questions.

- Was the restlessness recognised and correctly diagnosed?
- How was it managed?
- Were the interventions effective?

Read this chapter and decide whether you would now approach the situation differently.

What is terminal restlessness

The terms 'terminal restlessness', 'terminal anguish' and 'delirium' are often used interchangeably. Terminal restlessness overlaps with but is not necessarily identical to delirium.[1]

Terminal restlessness can be defined as the agitation and restlessness that may occur during the last few hours or days of life, and can be accompanied by any of the following:

- anxiety;
- impaired consciousness;
- myoclonus (muscular jerking).[2]

It occurs in approximately 42% of dying patients.[3]

Delirium – also known as acute confusional state – may be accompanied by:

- poor concentration;
- short-term memory loss;

- disorientation;
- paranoia;
- hallucinations;
- restlessness;
- noisy, aggressive behaviour.[4]

Confusion has already been covered in Chapter 2 on symptom control.

Assessment and goal

Assessment is the key to providing a safe, effective outcome in terminal restlessness. It is continuous, and not a 'one-off' process. The *goal* is as follows:

- to provide physical and emotional comfort;
- to maintain a conscious level that will enable family relationships and communication to continue for as long as possible;
- to reduce the distress of the relative(s).

Terminal restlessness is very distressing for both the patient and their relative(s), and it can easily be mismanaged due to fear of over-sedation. Therefore, skilled assessment and effective therapeutic intervention by the multidisciplinary team will maximise symptom control.

Identifying the cause

The causative factors leading to terminal restlessness need to be identified quickly and effectively. Only when a treatable cause has been identified can steps be taken to reduce or eliminate the symptoms (see Box 7.1).[2]

Box 7.1:   Treatable causes of terminal restlessness[2]

- Generalised physical discomfort.
- Bladder or bowel distension.
- Breathlessness.
- Anoxia.
- Nicotine withdrawal – use nicotine patch or Nicorette nasal spray.
- Alcohol withdrawal – use diazepam in decreasing doses for 7–10 days.
- Illicit drug withdrawal.
- Infection.
- Drug induced (e.g. antibiotics, anticonvulsants, digoxin, diuretics, non-steroidal anti-inflammatory drugs (NSAIDs), steroids, opioids or hypnotics).
- Dehydration.

If time allows, the cause should be identified and treated.[1] Pain should be excluded as a cause and will require appropriate analgesics (*see* Chapter 1).[1] About 40% of patients experience an exacerbation of pain at the end of life.[3]

When assessing terminal restlessness, the following factors should be considered.

- The cause may be multifactorial or it may not be found.[1]
- The cause is discovered in less than 50% of patients.[5]
- When the cause is found, it is often irreversible (e.g. liver failure or cerebral metastases).[1]
- It is often inappropriate to undertake tests if time is short or the patient is at home.
- The patient may be unable to state the cause of the restlessness (e.g. feeling uncomfortable, experiencing pain, feeling afraid).

Other causes of terminal restlessness are listed in Box 7.2.[2]

Box 7.2:   Other causes of terminal restlessness[2]

- Cerebral oedema.
- Heart failure.
- Primary brain tumour.
- Cerebral vascular accident (CVA).
- Biochemical imbalance (urea, calcium, sodium, glucose).
- Deteriorating liver and renal function.
- Unresolved psychosocial issues.

As well as assessing and correcting the cause of terminal restlessness or delirium, symptomatic and supportive measures are important for minimising the distress caused to the patient.[6] The opportunity should be taken to review all medication and, where necessary, to discontinue medication if appropriate.

Management

Pharmacological therapy and psychological intervention to minimise the distress of the patient and relative(s) are the mainstay of treatment for terminal restlessness. Practical support can include the following measures.

- Provide a safe environment. If the patient is delirious, there may be a danger to self and others.
- If appropriate, a mattress placed on the floor, although not ideal, may be a safer option in the acute situation.[7]
- Try to encourage a peaceful, quiet environment.

- Make full use of soft lighting. Fears are often exacerbated at night, and therefore a low light should be used at night to promote a feeling of safety.
- If appropriate, reassure the patient that someone will stay with them at all times. A member of the family or a familiar friend will help ro reduce distress. It is preferable to maintain continuity of care.[7]
- Gentle massage using relaxing essential oils may help to induce relaxation and maximise feelings of well-being. Essential oils, used in a vaporising burner, may both provide sensory pleasure and help to reduce anxiety.
- Touch can be powerful. It alerts the patient to your presence and demonstrates a feeling of care.
- Give simple and clear explanations of what is going to happen and what can be done to help the patient and their relative(s).
- It is important to reassure the relative(s) that terminal restlessness is often part of the process of dying. The relative(s) may feel responsible for the patient's symptoms – a sense that they have 'done something wrong'.[2]
- Ensure that the relative(s) have the opportunity for rest and time to themselves.
- An increased level of nursing supervision is essential.
- Make staff continuity a priority.

Cognitive interventions can apply to both the patient and their relative(s),[8] and can include the following:

- acknowledgement of the patient' feelings;
- alleviating isolation;
- fostering a sense of control;
- balancing hope and reality.

Pharmacological therapy

Key tip
Intramuscular (IM) injections are too painful for thin, frail patients, and should be avoided whenever possible in palliative care. The subcutaneous route is kinder and just as effective.

Many patients are unable to take oral medication due to their agitated state, fluctuating levels of consciousness or general level of debility.[9] Therefore the subcutaneous (*see* Chapter 3) or rectal route should be used in such cases.

The medication of choice for terminal restlessness *without* delirium is midazolam (a benzodiazepine).[1] The suggested dose range of midazolam is 30–100 mg per 24 hours via continuous subcutaneous infusion (for more information on continuous subcutaneous infusion, *see* Chapter 3).[9,10] It is important to remember to administer a stat.

dose of midazolam, 5 mg to 10 mg subcutaneously, prior to setting up the syringe driver. This will calm the agitated patient while the syringe driver medication is taking effect. Box 7.3 provides an 'at a glance' view of this treatment regime.

Box 7.3: Medication for terminal restlessness

Midazolam

Suggested range:[9,10]   30 mg to 100 mg p/24 hours via continuous subcutaneous infusion.

Stat. dose: 5 mg to 10 mg subcutaneously will help to calm the agitated patient whilst syringe-driver medication takes effect.

Levomepromazine

Suggested range:[3,14]   50 mg to 75 mg p/24 hours via continuous subcutaneous infusion.

Stat. dose: 25 mg subcutaneously.

Usual maximum dose: 300 mg/24 hours, occasionally more.

Midazolam

Midazolam, supplied as 5 mg in 1-mL ampoules, has a quick-onset action. It is water-soluble and mixes with most of the drugs that are commonly given by syringe driver.[4] In agitated terminal delirium, larger doses are sometimes necessary, especially if anxiety has been a feature, or in the case of a patient who has been using denial as a coping mechanism.[4] Tolerance may develop after the patient has shown a good initial response. Therefore continual review and dose increases, as necessary, are acceptable practice.[9]

Limitations

Midazolam has several disadvantages that must be borne in mind. Large volumes of the injection are needed when using a high dose. Therefore it is useful to use a larger syringe. A 20-mL or 30-mL syringe will fit Graseby pumps MS16[A] and MS26 (*see* Chapter 3). The syringe can be changed 6-, 8- or 12-hourly instead of 24-hourly,[9] if necessary.

Diazepam (a benzodiazepine)

Diazepam, given as a suppository per rectum (PR) is useful in a crisis.[4] A stat. dose of 20 mg, PR and 6- to 8-hourly, may be helpful in such cases.

Limitations

Rectal administration of diazepam at home may be difficult due to the practical problems of moving and changing position. It can only be used if the patient has given their consent (patients choice). There may be problems if the patient is impacted or has diarrhoea. Haemorrhoids, tumour, rectal discharge or pain may also exclude this route.[10,11]

Levomepromazine (methotrimeprazine – a phenothiazine)

Levomepromazine is often used to control agitation and confusion.[12] A stat. dose of 25 mg subcutaneously and 50 to 75 mg per 24 hours administered via a syringe driver may be beneficial. Titrate the dose, depending on the response. The usual maximum dose is 300 mg per 24 hours, and occasionally more.[13,14] The above treatment regime is illustrated in Box 7.3, which provides an 'at a glance' view. The onset of the drug action is approximately 30 minutes, and the duration of the dose action is 12–24 hours.[15] Levomepromazine can be advantageous because of its anti-emetic and analgesic benefits.[15] Levomepromazine is available in 25-mg tablets or as 25 mg in a 1 mL injection. If there is a risk of convulsions, midazolam, 30 to 60 mg per 24 hours, can be added.[4]

Haloperidol (a butyrophenone)

Haloperidol is the drug of choice for restlessness *with* delirium.[16,17] In low doses of 1 mg to 3 mg, it is usually effective in targeting the following:

- fear;
- agitation;
- paranoia.[1]

Oral haloperidol is effective, and some patients can be managed well with this.[1] Parenteral doses are approximately twice as potent as the equivalent oral dose.[1] Haloperidol can be administered over a 24-hour period via a syringe driver. Doses do not generally exceed 20 mg over 24 hours.[1]

The suggested range of Haloperidol is as follows:[15]

- in the elderly, 1.3 to 3 mg stat., and at night (nocte);
- in the younger patient, 5 mg stat., and at night (nocte);
- in cases of poor response, 10 to 30 mg at night (nocte), or in a divided dose.[15]

It is beneficial to titrate the drug to the behaviour.

It is acknowledged that haloperidol is useful for controlling agitation and improving cognition. However, if death is likely to occur soon, this may not be achievable.[1] The causes of delirium may be irreversible in the active, dying phase.[1] If the delirium cannot be reversed, sometimes it may be necessary to use the following:

- midazolam;
- levomepromazine.

So far, this chapter has concentrated on pharmacological intervention. However, it is important to remember the need for psychological intervention.

Psychological interventions

Although pharmacological intervention is the mainstay of the control of restlessness, agitation and delirium, it is important to be aware that psychological support is pivotal in helping to alleviate anxiety and distress. It is essential in the provision of a holistic and eclectic approach.

Unresolved emotions issues

Restlessness and agitation can be caused by unresolved issues in the patient's life. Spiritual pain or fear can be most resistant of all to treatment interventions.[2] Spiritual or emotional pain, fear and anger can be withheld from the community professional and may not be exposed until physical symptoms (e.g. pain, nausea, vomiting) are effectively controlled.

Whenever possible, emotional issues should be addressed early on with the patient, and also if appropriate – and with the patient's agreement – with their family. The family should be given the opportunity to discuss their own fears and concerns, away from the patient, thus addressing their own needs, which may be different to the needs of the patient. Ensuring that the environment is safe for such disclosure is essential and it may be necessary to arrange meetings within or outwith the patient's and/or relatives' home environment. It is important to make it clear that this is possible and can be arranged without problem.

In an attempt to ease spiritual and emotional distress, eclectic and holistic approaches to care can be utilised and, where appropriate, referral to other professionals and agencies, such as the following, should be made:

- counsellor;
- clinical psychologist;
- family therapist;
- religious leader.

Some individuals can never accept the fact that they are dying. Denial can be a means of coping right to the end of life. While supporting the patient and identifying and aiming to reduce distress, it is important that there is respect for the individual's choice. The patient needs to feel safe and have the opportunity to cope in whatever way is appropriate for them. This freedom of choice should be acknowledged by the professional at all times. However, there is a danger that if emotional distress is not addressed, the patient will often be unable to control the thoughts and unresolved fears that can break through into the confused mind with devastating results.[4]

Supporting the family

Guiding the family and demonstrating empathy by 'being with them' through this distressing time is an essential part of holistic and eclectic care. There are no short cuts. Teamwork is vital. Families benefit from a multidisciplinary approach that supports the many and varied needs of each individual. The family often experiences a sense of helplessness and isolation. They may feel that they are being pushed away by the patient. It needs to be acknowledged that as the 'professional' it is difficult for us, too, when we come across situations where we feel helpless. Therefore one can observe and appreciate that, for the family at such times, there is a constant reminder, sustained over many weeks or months that can, if it goes unrecognised, have a detrimental long-term effect on their lives.

It is important that the issues of sedation are discussed with the family. Their views are important and should always be taken into account. The community professional should aim to offer clear, straightforward information. Check the relatives' understanding throughout, and make sure that the family understand that the medication will make the patient feel sleepy, rendering verbal communication difficult. It is also just as important to listen to what is said and what is not said, giving time and opportunity for each family member to express their own individual concerns and the issues that are important to them.

Caring for themselves

Reassure the family that time set aside for them is important and that it is acceptable to take that time. Taking care of oneself is pivotal in enabling the care of the patient. Families often feel guilty about spending time on themselves. There is the feeling that 'personal time' can take them away from what they perceive they should be doing (i.e. looking after the patient).

Using supportive complementary therapies (e.g. a massage), relaxation techniques, and attending a support group, may be both possible and appropriate. Agencies within the family's local community may provide 'home carers,' who can stay with the patient while the family member shops, visits the hairdressers or attends to their own healthcare needs.

Aiming to be honest

Agreeing with the frightened, dying patient that they will get better and 'everything will be alright' is not necessarily helpful. It is easy for the family and the community professional to collude with the patient when they are unsure about what to say or do. Colluding may serve to undervalue their feelings, and blocks any useful communication, thus making 'letting go' difficult.

Listen carefully to their fears, concerns and questions. Watch for non-verbal communication, and be calm and genuine. Be yourself. Show that you understand, and that you are there – be with them. This is therapeutic in itself. Clever words and phrases are both inappropriate and unnecessary in such situations. The unspoken, the silence and the 'being with' can all offer comfort to the dying person.

Sometimes the patient needs to be 'given permission' to die by the family. People often wish to hold on to what they know and love. It can be a struggle for both parties to let go. It is sometimes sufficient for the family to tell the patient that it is all right for them to die.[18]

Dying may give rise to many repressed emotions, sadness, numbness, guilt, and jealousy of those who are well.[19] It is often helpful to the family for them to understand that being open and honest with the patient can open up channels of communication. This may be helped by facilitation by an appropriate professional. Often merely asking the patient 'how' they, the family, can help may be useful. The patient is sometimes able to give the family help and guidance in meeting their needs.

Conclusion

Terminal restlessness and agitation, with or without delirium, is a frightening experience for the patient, family and community professional, and it represents a challenge for the multidisciplinary team. Ongoing assessment and evaluation are central to achieving effective outcomes. Constant monitoring, using a team approach, is needed to enable rapid, effective and therapeutic responses to any change.

Preparing the family for the possible occurrence of restlessness and agitation may be a possibility. Reassurance that in most cases something can be done will help to reduce some of their inevitable anxieties, and is essential. Being prepared for possible events leading up to the patient's death may help the patient and their family to cope better with the events as and when they occur. If the family have some awareness and understanding that such events are sometimes part of dying, and not due to negligence in the care given to the patient, this may make it easier to talk the issue through with other relative(s) and help to minimise the extreme distress and difficulties that can occur in such situations.

Dying is not always peaceful. Although it should always be the aim of the community professional, realistically it is not always possible. It is of equal importance that, as community professionals, we take care of both our own needs and the needs of colleagues with whom we work. This topic will be addressed further in Chapters 14 and 15.

The following are essential for effective therapeutic intervention.

- Be clear about what can realistically be achieved.
- Use eclectic and holistic approaches to identified needs and problems.
- Keep up to date with current research and practice.
- Maximise the use of skills and knowledge (both intuitive and factual).

Being aware of the above will enable the community professional to provide the best possible care and to maximise support for the patient and their relative(s). Remember that both pharmacological and non-pharmacological therapies play an important role in the management of terminal restlessness in palliative care.

Patients and their relatives are real people facing real problems and traumatic situations, often with limited resources of their own. As health and social care professionals, we must respect each of them as an individual. Time should be taken at all stages to listen to what they say and also what they do not say, so that we can act to provide the highest standard of care and expertise that is available. It is imperative that we listen to these people as individuals, for they are the true experts.

Chapter 7: Questions

1 How would you define terminal restlessness?
2 List three possible treatable causes of terminal restlessness.
3 What practical support can be given to the patient?
4 What is the drug of choice for terminal restlessness without delirium?
5 What is the drug of choice for terminal restlessness with delirium?
6 List three emotions that may be repressed by the dying person.
7 What support can you give to the family and/or carer during this difficult time?

References

1   Breitbart W, Chochinovov HM and Passik S (1998) Psychiatric aspects of palliative care. In: D Doyle, GWC Hanks and N MacDonald (eds) *Oxford Textbook of Palliative Medicine* (2e). Oxford University Press, Oxford.

2   March PA (1998) Hospice techniques: terminal restlessness. *Am J Hospice Palliative Care.* **Jan/Feb:** 51–3.

3   Enck RE (1992) The last few days. *Am J Hospice Palliative Care.* 9: 11–13.

4   Twycross R (1997) *Symptom Management in Advanced Cancer* (2e). Radcliffe Medical Press, Oxford.

5 Bruera E, Miller L, McCallion J *et al.* (1992) Cognitive failure in patients with terminal cancer: a prospective study. *J Pain Symptom Management.* **7**: 192–5.

6 Lipowski ZJ (1987) Delirium (acute confusional state). *JAMA.* **285**: 1789–92.

7 Macleod AD (1997) The management of delirium in hospice practice. *Eur J Palliative Care.* **4**: 116–200.

8 Richeimer SH (1987) Psychological intervention in delirium. *Postgrad Med.* **81**: 173–80.

9 Bottomley DM and Hanks GW (1990) Subcutaneous midazolam infusion in palliative care. *J Pain Symptom Management.* **5**: 259–61.

10 De Sousa E and Jepson BA (1988) Midazolam in terminal care. *Lancet.* **i**: 67–8.

11 Amesbury BDW and Dunphy KP (1989) The use of subcutaneous midazolam in the home care setting. *Palliative Med.* **3**: 299–301.

12 Oliver DJ (1985) The use of methotrimeprazine in terminal care. *Br J Clin Practice.* **39**: 339–40.

13 Johnson I and Patterson S (1992) Drugs used in combination in the syringe driver: a survey of hospice practice. *Palliative Med.* **6**: 125–30.

14 Regnard CFB and Tempest S (1998) *A Guide to Symptom Relief in Advanced Disease* (4e). Hochland and Hochland, Manchester.

15 Twycross R, Wilcock A and Thorp S (1998) *PCF1 Palliative Care Formulary.* Radcliffe Medical Press, Oxford.

16 Taylor D and Lewis S (1993) Delirium. *J Neurosurg Psychiatry.* **5556**: 742–51.

17 Adams F, Fernandaz F and Andersson BS (1986) Emergency pharmacotherapy of delirium in the critically ill cancer patient. *Psychosomatics.* **27**: 33–7.

18 Callahan C and Kelly P (1992) *Final Gifts.* Poseidon Press, New York.

19 Rinpoche S (1998) *The Tibetan Book of Living and Dying.* Ryder, London.

To learn more

Callahan C and Kelly P (1992) *Final Gifts.* Poseidon Press, New York.

Doyle D, Hanks GW and MacDonald N (1998) *Oxford Textbook of Palliative Medicine.* Oxford University Press, Oxford.

McMahon R and Pearson A (1992) *Nursing as Therapy.* Chapman and Hall, London.

Rinpoche S (1998) *The Tibetan Book of Living and Dying.* Rider, London.

Twycross R (1997) *Symptom Management in Advanced Cancer* (2e). Radcliffe Medical Press, Oxford.

Twycross R, Wilcock A and Thorp S (1998) *PCF1 Palliative Care Formulary.* Radcliffe Medical Press, Oxford.

Chapter 7:   Answers

1 The agitation and restlessness that may occur in the last few hours or days of life.
2
  • Physical discomfort
  • Bladder or bowel distension
  • Breathlessness
  • Anoxia
  • Nicotine withdrawal
  • Alcohol withdrawal
  • Illicit drug withdrawal
  • Infection
  • Other drugs
  • Dehydration.

3
  • Provision of a safe environment
  • A mattress on the floor
  • A peaceful, quiet environment
  • Use of soft lighting, with low lights at night
  • Continuity of carers and a familiar friend or family member to stay with the patient
  • Gentle massage with relaxing oils
  • Appropriate use of touch
  • Providing information and an explanation to the family.

4 Midazolam.
5 Haloperidol.
6 Sadness, numbness, guilt, jealousy of those who are well.
7 Now that you have read this chapter you may be able to think of other approaches you could use. The important thing to remember is to be yourself and to be genuine in your responses.

PART TWO

Practical approaches to the needs of the individual

CHAPTER 8

Hearing the pain of the carer

Mandy Redgrove and Audrey Smyth

Case scenario

Tom is facing a life-threatening illness. He has cancer, and although his family, friends and colleagues do not, *they too are facing this disease*. All of them, Tom's child, grandchild, partner and friends, are confronted with death, fear and loss, and for Tom and everyone in his world, life has changed.

Introduction

In this chapter you are invited to explore how, in the work you do, you might help the people who relate in one way or another to a person like Tom. The chapter aims to share knowledge and experience gained from listening to many people who are close to someone with a life-threatening disease, how a person in this position might feel, what they might need, and what is necessary for you to go at least some way towards meeting that need.

This chapter is based on the experiences of the authors as therapists in health and social work settings.

Who is 'the carer'?

The term 'carer' may not always be acceptable because it tends to be associated with a patient's *physical care*. Therefore it is important to be aware of Tom as more than a physical being. Only then does the notion of caring broaden. The carer is someone who, through a relationship with Tom, can recognise his value as a human being and so restore his spirit and sense of self-worth. For the purpose of this chapter, the 'carer' will be referred to as Mary. However, this could describe *anyone*, of either sex and any relationship who is significant to Tom, including young adults and children.

Who is suffering?

Quite often (in fact, usually) Mary will say 'what have I got to complain about? After all, it's Tom who is ill and facing his death, he must come first'. Tom may well return home from having treatment at the hospital and say 'you know, I ought to be thankful. A person I met in the hospital was having a *much* worse time than me, poor thing.'

This tendency to see pain and suffering *relatively* may be a way of trying to minimise it in order to make it a little more bearable. Although it is always possible to find another human being who can be perceived as being worse off, in the end these comparisons provide no lasting comfort.

When working with carers it is important not to collude with their trivialisation of the pain and suffering they inevitably experience. It is much healthier for the carer to be given room and encouragement to express what is *really* going on inside – the fears, frustration and helplessness.

So in answer to the question 'who is suffering?', it could be suggested that it is *Tom and all those around him*. Suffering is suffering. There is no pecking order, and everyone's needs count. This approach fosters the idea that Tom and Mary can come together in an equal, open, reciprocal relationship, rather than Mary martyring herself and making it impossible for Tom to give anything to her. It is precisely that situation which would lead to Tom feeling isolated, redundant and a burden, and Mary feeling trapped and unable to acknowledge her own feelings and needs.

What might the carer feel?

It is very likely that Mary will feel a need to be strong and positive for Tom. She will feel responsible for keeping him and his hope alive. It is also likely that she herself does not dare to contemplate the possibility that he might die. Even if she does acknowledge this, the prospect may be frightening.

Mary could be facing a spiritual crisis of her own. It is possible that she has not faced her own mortality and that she finds it disturbing. In turn, she will avoid Tom's need to address his death, his suffering and what his life has meant. This drives a wedge of unease and discomfort between them, and both are left floundering alone in spiritual distress.

Mary feels lost and isolated. Due to Tom's 'protection' of her and her own 'protection' of him, communication in any meaningful sense ceases. She feels that the relationship with Tom has been lost. Indeed, if the relationship has been a physically intimate one, this emotional distance may well be mirrored in a lack of physical and sexual contact. The sexual relationship may be further complicated if the disease has affected Tom's physical appearance, his body image and his mobility. Mary may feel emotionally and physically distant at the very time when she and Tom need each other most.

In this sea of uncertainty and isolation, it is understandable that Mary may become self-doubting and unsure about how to 'get it right' for Tom. People speak of a feeling of 'treading on eggshells', of being fearful of speaking about anything important – like the diagnosis, the future or what to tell the children. The fear is that to speak of such things might make everything worse.

The stress and tension that result from bottling up all of these feelings often give rise to anger and an acute sense of helplessness. Many people have described how they have expressed this frustration by being short-tempered, and subsequently have felt guilty, particularly when their anger has been directed at their dying relative.

Often Mary will feel a tremendous responsibility for Tom's physical well-being and treatment. There are countless decisions to be made about when and where to seek medical attention, how to obtain information, which treatment option to pursue, and even what Tom should eat. Trying to make such decisions can place a tremendous strain on the relationship.

These responsibilities are in addition to any physical nursing that has to be done. Exhaustion is common, and is often followed by a feeling of failure and inability to cope. What at first seems like the obvious solution – handing over to someone else – is fraught with difficulty. Mary, understandably, may not want to relinquish her role to someone who will not be able to care for Tom in the way that she does. There is no respite if Mary is consumed with anxiety and sadness whenever she is away from Tom. In addition, it is common for patients like Tom to want only the person they know intimately to care for them. It may be the only way in which physical contact between them is possible, impacting on their sexuality and the potential loss of sexual function.

Many of the feelings experienced by adult carers are also felt by young adults and children. Their situation can be made worse by adults, who, by attempting to protect them, often exclude them from the reality of an illness. Such seclusion increases anxiety and helplessness. This chapter is concerned with how you can support an adult carer, but the concept is just as relevant to the young adult and child. However, different skills are needed to communicate with young adults and children. If you do not have the necessary experience, then it is essential that support for the young adult or child is found elsewhere.

What might the carer need?

Mary is facing a painful experience. Tom, whom she loves, is ill with a life-threatening disease. What does she need? And what might she do to cope with her

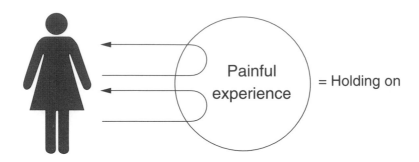

Figure 8.1   Coping by self-distraction and avoiding feelings.

situation? When something triggers her feeling of fear and loneliness, she will probably try to avoid this pain by self-distraction and pulling away from what she feels. She may do this by concentrating on the need to be 'strong' for Tom, by keeping busy, or by watching television. Most of us know these 'coping' strategies, and sometimes they are necessary and useful for getting through the practicalities of daily life.

This scenario can be seen more clearly in Figure 8.1. The arrows represent Mary repeatedly touching the painful experience and then pulling away from it. She avoids feelings, sometimes for practical reasons, but more often because she fears that if she starts crying she will never stop, and that she might 'crack up' and be of no use to anyone. In Figure 8.1 there is no sense of *movement*, except round in circles. Indeed, there is a sense of *holding on to* the pain, almost of *closing around it* in fear.

In Figure 8.2 rather than Mary recoiling from her experience, she allows herself to feel it completely. There is a sense of movement *through* these feelings, and of release and relief. For this to happen, Mary needs the support of a relationship with someone who is unafraid of her 'negative' feelings, who is able to 'hold' her through them and who is confident of the healing power of their expression. Such a relationship

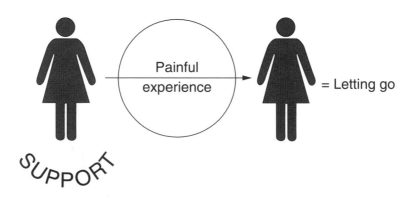

Figure 8.2   Coping by expression of 'negative' feelings.

provides Mary with the encouragement, permission and safety to let go of what she feels.*

The establishment of this accepting, supporting relationship is absolutely fundamental to the work you do to accompany someone in Mary's position through this turbulent time.

Many issues will come up for her. Examples might include the following.

- Why is this happening to us?
- What do I believe in?
- What is death?
- Should I give up work?
- How will we manage financially?
- What should we tell the children?
- How can I talk to Tom about dying?
- What about making a will and arranging a funeral?
- How can I support Tom when he goes to see the consultant?
- What treatments should Tom opt for?
- What if Tom loses hope and feels despair?
- What if Tom is in pain?

By listening and helping Mary to explore these issues, you provide her with an opportunity to see the whole situation, including her part in it, more clearly. She will feel steadier and less agitated. As a result of her work with you, she is more likely to enjoy an open and honest relationship with Tom where difficulties and feelings are shared and unfinished business is dealt with. Helping Mary to use this limited time as effectively as possible means that she and Tom will experience a richer relationship. It will also prevent her from having to live with regrets after Tom has died. *In essence, what Mary really needs is for you to enter her world and be alongside her.*

Mary will need knowledge of organisations which can provide her with information, services and practical resources. There are organisations which operate nationally. It is advisable to find out about any local services (such as the hospice) which could offer staff support, equipment, respite and therapies.

What does it take for you, the worker, to support the carer?

To answer this question, you will probably consider what you could *do* to support the carer. Yet, if you look at your own experience of being well supported, it is likely to have been as much to do with *how* that person behaved towards you as to anything they may have done practically.

---

*This model was shared with us by Bill Sandhu, a dear friend who taught us most of what we know about working alongside people.

So what it does take to support Mary? You, the worker, need to be *open-hearted and touched by her experience*. This requires that you can simply accept and 'sit with' her feelings, however painful they may be. In this way, you can be sensitive to and *really hear* what Mary's world is like. As a result, your responses are likely to be spontaneous, natural and helpful. You will be less likely to put yourself under pressure and find instant solutions, give advice or tell her what to do. Instead, you will offer her a relationship within which she can find her own way and make her own decisions. This does not mean sitting passively, doing nothing. In fact, to support Mary well, you may need to challenge her. You may also need to take risks by asking direct questions about sensitive issues.

Awareness of what might prevent you from offering Mary this supportive relationship is important. Avoidance of your own pain and fears can lead you to close your ears and heart to her suffering. There are many ways of distancing yourself, all of which are unhelpful. One of them is to present yourself as an 'invincible' professional helper. In doing this, you cast Mary in the role of 'the helpless'. This merely serves to protect you and disempower her.

It is imperative to attend to your own personal growth. This includes addressing your own death and spirituality. It is not a matter of religion, or knowing all the answers to what is often a mystery. Supervision, therapy and spiritual practices can be helpful – basically whatever is right for you. *When you are doing this work, it is important to look after yourself.*

Conclusion

Having faith in yourself and the confidence to simply be human, rather than an expert who 'knows it all', is the key to supporting the carer. It sounds so easy, but in reality it requires continual self-searching and openness. It is more demanding than learning a set of skills. However, as human beings we have an innate capacity to love and be compassionate. It is a question of uncovering what is already there inside us all.

Reflective exercise

Take time to reflect on what you have read in this chapter. Has it helped to raise your awareness of the needs of the carer? Has it increased your awareness of your own needs? Take a few minutes to write down your thoughts.

To learn more

Brewin T (1996) *Relating to the Relatives: Breaking Bad News, Communication and Support.* Radcliffe Medical Press, Oxford.

Dass R and Gorman P (1985) *How Can I Help?* Century, London.

Levine S (1987) *Healing into Life and Death.* Gateway Books, Bath.

Longaker C (1997) *Facing Death and Finding Hope: A Guide to the Emotional and Spiritual Care of the Dying.* Century, London.

Siegel B (19930 *Living, Loving and Healing.* HarperCollins, London.

CHAPTER 9

Spirituality: sharing the journey

Rosemary Booth

Are you afraid of spirituality? *Please don't be.*

Pre-reading exercise

Before reading this chapter, spend a few moments reflecting on your own understanding of spirituality.
Does your work involve concern for the spirit?

Spirituality is an integral part of palliative care and influences every aspect of it. Significant for all human beings, spirituality is about absolutely anything which relates to the spirit. It is not confined to people who have a religious belief. Issues of spirituality are wide-ranging and include questions about meaning and purpose in life, the search for hope, attitudes to other people, approaches to caring for and being with people, and the relationships which affect us all. Paying attention to spirituality is important for both patient and carer, and has difficult as well as beneficial aspects. This chapter suggests how the experience can be enriching for all concerned.

Many everyday things can 'lift the spirit':

- a beautiful view; a glorious sunset; inspiring music, art or poetry;
- a gift of flowers, a letter or a visit from a friend;
- a prayer for healing; an expression of love and support; a smile or a hug;
- a delicious meal or a glass of wine; lightheartedness; a good joke.

By contrast, the spirit can be crushed by so much that is encountered in everyday life:

- insensitivity; unkind or thoughtless words; lack of love;
- rough handling; aggressive behaviour or body language;
- dreary surroundings; isolation; loneliness; feeling unloved or rejected.

Meaning and purpose

The challenge of serious illness and the possibility of death often lead to the questioning of long-held beliefs and ideas. Looking back and reviewing life events may result in resentment or bitterness, or perhaps the realisation that time is short and that broken relationships need to be resolved. Regret or guilt about past behaviour may prompt the desire for forgiveness. Alienation from other people or from God, and also feelings of unworthiness, are powerful factors that require attention before peace of mind can be achieved. Searching for meaning and purpose in all that has happened to a person may be something only that person can do. During the process, sensitive listening is needed.

Encouraging hope

The concept of hope can seem futile in palliative care, but it is very significant to patients and their families. Perhaps long-term hope in the future may be unrealistic, but the setting of small, achievable goals does a great deal to encourage hopefulness in everyday life.

The following are some examples.

- Effective pain control and a good night's sleep improve quality of life.
- Being able to get dressed raises self-esteem.
- Imaginative food preparation and the use of anti-emetics make enjoyment of a meal possible.
- Leaving the home for a short outing is stimulating.
- Recalling past experiences or relationships which were happy and satisfying helps to boost confidence in dealing with current difficulties.
- Simple explanations about the illness or treatment can alleviate anxiety.
- The availability of symptom control and the reassurance of continuing support reduce fear and promote hope.

Identifying spiritual distress – what is needed?

To begin with, a calm, sensitive approach and good listening skills are needed. Giving full attention to the person concerned is an effective way of conveying

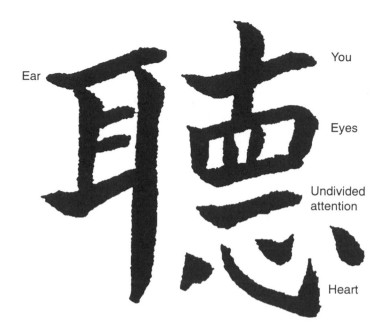

Figure 9.1 Chinese character for listening.

interest and a desire to help. Initially, ways of affirming your interest might include the following:

- taking off your outdoor coat;
- accepting the offer of a cup of tea;
- sitting down, being still, and making eye contact;
- avoiding chatter, but initiating a conversation in which the patient's own agenda has priority.

This kind of approach helps to establish a trusting relationship. It implies a concern about the whole person, not just about physical comfort, medication and practical matters. Most people will gladly accept the rare opportunity to have a listener's undivided attention.

Quiet observation of the patient is necessary. It may be obvious that fear or anxiety is present. Facial expression or body language often provide some indication of mental state. Encouraging the person to talk about what has been happening to them – to tell their story – will give them the opportunity to identify experiences, fears or anxieties that are troubling them. Sometimes strong emotion will be expressed. Anger, fear, jealousy, anguish, regret and guilt can seem overwhelming to both patient and listener. Absorbing another person's emotion is hazardous and it may be damaging. Too much can lead to burnout and exhaustion. Understanding and an awareness of yourself and your own need for support help to safeguard against such difficulties.

Listening – the heart of spirituality

Listening is at the heart of spirituality. It requires the response of the whole person. This is well illustrated by the Chinese character for listening (Figure 9.1). It means conveying a feeling of warmth, love and acceptance that enables the 'patient' to put his or her feelings into words. It often means not being afraid of silence. This is the time needed for searching for ideas and thoughts, developing a theme and deciding what to say. Most of us find it difficult to express our deepest thoughts and needs in times of health and well-being. In illness, everything is more difficult. Thoughts are confused, words take time to come to mind, and the slightest interruption can set back the flow of speech.

Seeking further help for the patient or family member

After careful listening and talking with the patient or family member, it will be possible to identify one or more issues that need further attention. Sometimes the help which is needed can be provided by you, but issues which are complex or of a specific nature may require the involvement of a particular type of specialist.

Sharing the load – the importance of teamwork

No one person should try to do everything in palliative care – teamwork is paramount. Facilitating the work of colleagues is vital and requires skill and self-confidence. There is a danger of becoming possessive about patient and family which may stem from insecurity and a lack of self-awareness. It is not in the best interests of those on the receiving end of care. However, drawing others into the team and giving a warm introduction facilitates the practice of others and gives confidence to the patient.

Establishing and leading a team so that the patient and their family can benefit from a wide range of skills and competencies is an art. Maintaining appropriate support for the team and facilitating contact between team members during the illness of the patient is a little like conducting an orchestra! It is hard work, and requires considerable emotional energy. Sometimes it is unclear exactly who is the leader of the orchestra, and in fact the leadership may change from time to time. Team meetings where thoughts and ideas can be shared on a regular basis may be considered time-consuming. However, they are essential as they help to ensure the best possible quality of care. They can also be very enjoyable, encouraging and supportive!

Qualities needed by the professional carer

Responding to the spiritual needs of another human being involves a kind of shared journey with that person. This demands an openness to the thoughts and ideas of other people as well as your own. It requires a willingness to learn new things, and a desire for personal growth and development. A certain amount of self-disclosure may be appropriate – this becomes possible and comfortable when one human being truly meets with another. Sharing in this way is not about relating a catalogue of our own problems. It acknowledges that learning is a two-way process and that something the patient has said affects you. Relating to each other as two human beings promotes rather than detracts from the therapeutic relationship. The concept of the wounded healer is significant here. However, risks are involved. Openness leads to a vulnerability that needs to be recognised. Discovering and practising a personal faith or philosophy of life is a significant part of the support system that is needed as much by the professional carer as by the sick person.

Religious belief

For many people religious belief has a special significance towards the end of life. Individual beliefs, faith and preferences need to be respected and provided for. It is impossible to know or understand about these without asking, and assumptions can be very dangerous! So, ask something along the following lines.

- Do you have a faith that is meaningful to you?
- Is there a religious leader you would like to see?

Asking the question gives the patient a choice. It also acknowledges a concern beyond the merely physical or practical.

A personal faith or religious belief may be a source of tremendous strength and support to a sick person. Making possible the practice of that faith is an important part of spirituality in palliative care. This may involve practical arrangements such as providing a quiet place for prayer. There may also be issues of distress that relate specifically to a person's religious belief which need attention. Examples of these might include the following:

- anger with God;
- feelings of sinfulness and guilt;
- fear about God's anger and possible punishment after death;
- alienation from other people, or feeling out of touch with God.

Sometimes all that is required is the simple assurance that God forgives. In other situations, it will be necessary to arrange a visit from a priest, minister or appropriate religious leader. Special sensitivity is needed when identifying and providing for the needs of minority groups. The availability of skilled help gives the patient and their family the best opportunity to resolve difficulties. The peace of mind that is likely to follow contributes greatly to the well-being of the patient.

Relationships

At the core of spirituality is the quality of the relationships which are forged between the patient, carers, family members, professional carers and the primary healthcare team.

Relationships with patient and family

Help and support may be needed to resolve and heal, where possible, broken or difficult relationships within the family. This is likely to be time-consuming and stressful. However, the relief of tension and anxiety that follows more than justifies the effort involved. This is of immense value to both the patient's well-being and to the well-being of the relatives who live on after the death and must deal with their bereavement.

Box 9.1:   Example Case 1: Facilitating communication

Dorothy and Betty were two friends who had lost contact due to changing circumstances and illness. Dorothy developed advanced cancer. When questioned about her main problem, Dorothy expressed concern about her friend. She was afraid that Betty, a stroke patient, who was no longer able to speak, might feel abandoned and neglected. Facilitating communication between these two friends, and providing transport so that a meeting between them could take place, brought great joy to both of them. Afterwards, Dorothy relaxed more easily and her symptom control seemed to be less difficult.

Relationships within the professional team

Working together as a team in the care of both patient and family brings great rewards. If the needs of the patient are to be addressed adequately, it is important for all team members to be relaxed and at ease with each other. This means that it must be possible for care strategies to be discussed within the team without individuals feeling threatened. Truly sharing ideas and feelings with one another leads to an optimum level of care for the patient and support for the family. In order to achieve this professionals need to relate to each other in the same way as they do to their patients, by:

- making time and expressing interest;
- sitting down, adopting a relaxed position and establishing eye contact;

- putting others at ease and making them comfortable;
- encouraging others to share thoughts and ideas;
- acknowledging the contributions and successes of others.

The importance of supervision

Supervision helps to maintain a balance for both the individual and the team. It is a tremendous asset in palliative care. Reviewing and reflecting on what has happened helps to make sense of things and provides a valuable learning opportunity. Team members have the opportunity to hear how others have reacted to demanding or emotional situations. Growth and development of both the individual and the team are encouraged.

Box 9.2:   Example Case 2: Team debriefing

Susan, a client in a local authority Day Centre, died. Members of staff and Susan's hospice nurse met to share their thoughts and feelings about her death. The occasion was simple and moving. It provided an opportunity for people to put into words ideas about death and dying, which they had never expressed before. This contributed to everyone's development. There was crying and laughter, and to conclude the meeting everyone joined in a group hug! Afterwards, people worked at a deeper level with each other and with their clients.

Practical aspects of spiritual care

So much that is said or done has an impact on the spirit. Spirituality is concerned with an approach to people – it is about a way of being with people.

Every human being who has ever been ill or in hospital is aware of the effect that the individual visitor (either professional or lay person) has on them. It is important that the patient feels better after the visit! The sensitive visitor avoids:

- staying too long – this leads to exhaustion;
- talking about their own personal problems;
- describing other peoples' illnesses and death;
- chattering about inconsequential matters;
- being afraid of silence. This is often the time needed for the patient to gather their thoughts and decide what they want to say. Interrupting or finishing a sentence for someone can be equally disastrous. It is so easy to get it wrong! Just as spaces are needed on a page to emphasise the words, so pauses and silences in a conversation are necessary to emphasise what is being said.

Nurturing the spirit

Surroundings have an impact, too. Pleasant surroundings are much appreciated and do a great deal to nurture the spirit. The patient's surroundings may be enhanced by:

- a bowl of fresh flowers;
- clean bed linen;
- an arrangement of family photographs;
- a comfortable chair for visitors.

All of these help to create an air of welcome, to soothe the spirit and promote peace and relaxation. Sometimes, in our rush to heal the body, we leave no time to heal the spirit, no time to listen and no time just to be with a person.

Box 9.3:   Example Case 3: Nurturing the spirit

Polly lived alone. Her brother came to visit her. There was little in the room to relieve the drabness of the surroundings. A nurse picked daisies from the grass outside and arranged them in an egg-cup on the table by her bed. A year after Polly's death, her brother remembered the daisies and recognised them as a sign of love and care.

Nurses will recall the guilty feeling they experienced – perhaps in their student days – when they stopped to talk with a patient. There was an ever present awareness that 'more important' things needed to be done. In fact, that brief encounter may have met the patient's greatest need at the time and been a very valuable part of his or her total care.

Time need not always be a constraint. A spiritual approach to care is not necessarily dependent on time. It is much more about the way in which people relate to each other with respect, love and understanding.

Reflective exercise

I hope that what you have just read will be of help in making spirituality meaningful in your work. Now try listing five ways in which your practice might change or be influenced as a result of reading this chapter.

To learn more

Dawson J (1994) *Spiritual Pain – in a Hospice Context*. St Columba's Fellowship, Windsor.

Frankl V (1987) *Man's Search for Meaning*. Hodder and Stoughton, London.

Keating K (1986) *The Little Book of Hugs*. Harper Collins, London.

Keating K (1988) *Second Little Book of Hugs*. Harper Collins, London.

Mud and Stars – The Impact of Hospice Experience on the Church's Ministry of Healing. Report of a Working Party on the impact of hospice experience on the Church's Ministry of Healing 1991–93. Sobell Publications, Oxford.

Narayanasamy B (1991) *Spiritual Care. A Resource Guide – a Practical Guide for Nurses*. Quay Publishing BKT Information Services, Lancaster/Nottingham.

Neuberger J (1987) *Caring for People of Different Faiths*. Lisa Sainsbury Foundation Series, London.

Nouwen H (1979) *The Wounded Healer*. Darton, Longman and Todd Ltd, London.

Saunders C (1990) *Beyond the Horizon – a Search for Meaning in Suffering*. Darton, Longman and Todd Ltd, London.

Siegel B (1993) *Living, Loving and Healing*. Harper Collins, London.

Speck P (1995) *Being There. Pastoral Care in Time of Illness*. SPCK, London.

Vanier J (1988) *The Broken Body – Journey to Wholeness*. Darton, Longman and Todd Ltd, London.

Wilcock P (1996) *Spiritual Care of Dying and Bereaved People*. SPCK, London.

CHAPTER 10

Bereavement

Jenny Penson

Pre-reading exercise

Before reading this chapter, take time to consider the following question.

• What kinds of loss are you aware of?

Take a few minutes to reflect on your own life, and then write these down.

Introduction

'The loss of a loved person is one of the most intensely painful experiences any human being can suffer, and not only is it painful to experience, but also painful to witness, if only because we're so impotent to help.'

These words of Bowlby's[1] speak to me both as a human being and as a nurse. For if we don't know how to help, the natural tendency is to avoid the situation. If we do avoid it, we are likely to feel guilty. Therefore, this chapter aims to *provide knowledge, enhance skills* and *encourage confidence* so that we can be helpful to people who are facing the challenge of bereavement.

Box 10.1: Self-assessment question

Loss, grief, mourning and bereavement are all terms frequently seen in the literature. Are they interchangeable? Do they really mean the same thing?

The essential concept is loss. We have all experienced losses in our lives. These include the expected losses that are inherent in any transition from one stage of life to another. They are part of any change even when it is one that brings many gains (e.g. marriage or the birth of a wanted child).

There are losses that are *hidden* or even invisible. Others may be unaware that the loss has occurred (e.g. miscarriage or abortion). It could be the death of a more distant family member such as a grandparent, aunt or uncle, or a special friend. Families from a first marriage may not feature in the everyday life of the families from a second one. Therefore, bereavement may not be acknowledged or support may not be forthcoming.

In our work, we are familiar with the *physical* losses that are part of many disease processes and – sometimes – of treatment. Cancer provides a pertinent example, often involving changes in body image caused by weight loss as well as by surgery, chemotherapy or radiation. Bereavement can be likened to the amputation of a limb, because many people feel that they have lost part of themselves when their loved one dies.

As nurses, we may have deliberately concealed a death out of misdirected kindness – perhaps by not telling other patients on a ward that someone has died, or by colluding in not telling a child that his parent is going to die until it is too late. Parkes[2] refers to these as *disenfranchised* losses. Maybe we need to question our motives by asking whom we are trying to protect. We may find that we are protecting ourselves as much as our patients and their families from the painful questions that may arise.

Box 10.2:   Self-assessment question

For many bereaved people major loss leads to *multiple* losses.
Can you think of some examples of these?

It may be helpful to group them under the following headings, seen here with some examples:

- physical losses – touch, intimacy, sexuality;
- emotional losses – sharing, support, affection;
- spiritual losses – crises of faith, changing values and beliefs;
- loss of personal identity – role, status;
- lifestyle – financial security, changed relationships with others;
- patterns of living – taking on new tasks, changing work, moving house.

Grief describes the response to loss. This is composed of a strong and sometimes overwhelming variety of emotions, including the following:

- shock;
- anger;
- guilt;

- despair;
- sadness;
- restlessness;
- anxiety.

These can render the bereaved person vulnerable to illness and even to death, although the evidence for this is not conclusive.[3-5] Grief is experienced physically with sensations such as shortness of breath, palpitations, indigestion, headaches, muscle tension or fatigue.

Mourning refers to society's response to loss – the behaviours and rituals that are considered appropriate in any particular community or country. The absence of prescribed ways of behaving in modern western society is considered to be detrimental to the bereavement process.[6]

Bereavement literally means *to be robbed of something valued*. This appears to be a helpful definition because the word 'rob' indicates that the person has been wrongfully taken away – they should not have died. Therefore there is a sense of injustice, which often gives rise to strong and overwhelming emotions. It refers to the situation of anyone who has lost a person to whom they were strongly attached.

Box 10.3: Self-assessment question

Think about a time when you felt some of the emotions of loss. Perhaps you failed an important examination, went for an interview but didn't get the job, moved to a new area and left all your friends behind, or maybe you had a much-loved pet that died. Many of us will have experienced the loss of someone close, either through death or through divorce or other kinds of separation.
What were some of the feelings you experienced then?

The following case study illustrates feelings that are commonly experienced in bereavement.

Case 10.1

Sylvia was a 60-year-old woman whose twin sons both lived abroad, although they were very supportive of their mother, telephoning her regularly and communicating via e-mail. She was with her husband John when he died peacefully in a hospice following a short illness. Feelings of shock, numbness and disbelief overcame her, although she had stayed with him for many days. All she could say was 'I just can't take it in'. For some weeks afterwards she felt she was 'on automatic pilot really', and later she could not remember much of what she had done or the people she had seen.

The pain of grief is often felt physically, with the symptoms which are familiar to us when we are stressed. For example, Sylvia complained of insomnia, lack of appetite, and a general restlessness which meant that she could not bear to sit still for long enough to watch her favourite television programmes.

She experienced periods of intense anxiety leading to shortness of breath and panic attacks. Until these were explained to her, she thought that she had also developed cancer of the lung, like her husband. Many bereaved people do complain of physical symptoms that are similar to those suffered by their loved one.

Next came the strong emotions of anger, which took Sylvia by surprise. Normally a mild and conciliatory person, she felt almost overwhelmed by the strength of the anger she felt. The targets for Sylvia's anger moved around her. She blamed God because her husband had lived what she called 'a blameless life'. He was tolerant and kind, and it was as if God had not kept his side of the bargain. She blamed the GP who did not send her husband for tests early enough. She blamed one of her sons for causing her husband financial worry, which led to him being stressed just before the cancer was diagnosed. She blamed herself for not insisting that he saw the GP earlier when his flu symptoms did not clear up, and for urging him to do heavy work in the garden before the winter when he still wasn't well. What made her feel even more guilty was that she was angry with him for leaving her before they could enjoy their retirement together. Guilt is seen as anger turned in one oneself.

Sylvia felt intensely lonely as she began to accept the reality that her husband would not return in this life. She experienced periods of searching, when she would catch sight of someone in a car park or at the supermarket and think that it was John. She told how on one occasion she had rushed through a crowded store in pursuit of someone who was wearing a similar jacket to her husband. 'Part of me knew that this was ridiculous', she explained, 'but I couldn't seem to stop myself. I really thought I must be losing my mind.' This led to despair and hopelessness, an apathy that made her reluctant to get up in the morning, to prepare a meal or to contemplate any kind of future. Friends tried to persuade her to go out, attend a charity lunch or join a theatre visit, but she felt unable to socialise, and when she did make the effort she often felt worse afterwards.

She was uncharacteristically disorganised, taking hours to get ready to go out, dialling telephone numbers and then hastily putting down the receiver because she had forgotten who she was telephoning. She experienced what Torrie[7] referred to as a 'see-saw of feelings', where one minute she yearned for company, and the next she wanted to be left alone. She found herself out shopping with odd coloured shoes on and did not know whether to laugh or cry. She went home and did both.

It was impossible to pinpoint when Sylvia began to recover. 'It wasn't one dramatic event or anything like that – it just seems, looking back, that I'm better now than I was then. I'm beginning to plan things a bit. I can go out and not panic. I feel dreadful sometimes, but I suppose I feel there's some hope.' C.S. Lewis[8] describes such a turning point in his own bereavement when he writes about a gradual feeling of hope and the possibility of moving forward in new directions.

There are many perspectives on the experience of bereavement. Some see it as an adaptive process,[1] while others view it as a psychosocial transition,[9] a series of tasks[10] or a major stress.[11] The consensus seems to be that the expression of grief in some form is essential in order to adjust to bereavement.

Box 10.4:   Self-assessment question

Does anticipatory grieving help the bereavement process?

Bereavement begins from the moment the relative knows that the patient is not going to recover. This is sometimes referred to as anticipatory grieving. It is often considered to be helpful to adjustment, contrasting with an unexpected death where there has been no opportunity to say goodbye, to resolve family issues or to ask or receive forgiveness.[12] However, another view is that anticipation of the death intensifies attachment to the dying person, rather than bringing about detachment.[13] Silverman[14] concluded that talking about impending death was not grieving in advance, and that this could only happen after the death had taken place. Sometimes grieving in advance can lead to treating the person as if they have already died. For some individuals, grieving can only begin after the person has died.

Box 10.5:   Self-assessment questions

What assessment of Sylvia's needs could you make?
Reflect and write down your own points before continuing with this chapter.

Information that may be helpful includes:

- age;
- state of health;
- relationship with her husband and others in the family;
- the kind of death (expected? peaceful?);
- where it took place (hospital? nursing home? at home?);
- presence at the time of death;
- social factors (financial situation, community support);
- information from those who were involved in her husband's care before and at the time of his death.

Box 10.6:   Key point

It may be helpful to devise a form for communicating so that the local hospital, hospice, nursing home and community staff have clear guidelines on the simplest and most effective form of liaison.

Box 10.7:   Self-assessment question

What questions could you ask?
Take a few moments to think before reading on.

Of course, there can never be a blueprint of what to say, because each person and situation is unique. Our purpose is to encourage the bereaved person to tell us 'their story'. The sensitive acknowledgment of their loss can be a helpful starting point. Questions that might help to elicit their perspectives and feelings might include the following.

- What is the worst thing for you at the moment?
- When are the low points?
- How do you handle the difficult times?
- What do you find helpful?
- How do you see things working out in the future?

Box 10.8:   Self-assessment question

What risk factors are you aware of that could lead to problems in adjustment during bereavement?
Make some notes before reading further.

These risk factors include the following:

- timeliness;
- death of a child;
- social isolation;
- ambivalent relationship;
- nature of the loss;
- sudden death.

The *timeliness* (or otherwise) of the loss is linked to the nature of the relationship. It is considered that the death of an elderly person is easier to grieve than that of a young one. Therefore the death of a child is the hardest loss to grieve, and this is true even when the 'child' is an older person being grieved over by an elderly parent.

Social isolation is a common factor, especially in the elderly. Although a few people seem to have deep inner resources and little need for contact, most of us need to be in a relationship with others in order to thrive.

All relationships carry with them a degree of *ambivalence*. However, in cases where there has been an insecure attachment to the deceased, or a relationship where one person has been overly dependent and the other very dominant, there may be particular problems in adjustment.

The *nature* of the loss includes factors to do with the type of relationship with the deceased, and whether the death was anticipated or unexpected. A death that occurred by violence, suicide or catastrophe will usually necessitate skilled help.

It is generally agreed that *sudden* death is the largest single risk factor in bereavement, as in this case there has been no opportunity to anticipate the loss in any way. There will be a strong sense of shock and the possibility of disagreements, conflicts or unresolved issues just prior to the death.

Risk assessment tools can help to identify who could benefit most from intervention. It appears that the majority of such tools are derived from the Bereavement Risk Index (BRI).[13]

Box 10.9:   Self-assessment question

Reflecting on the case study of Sylvia's experience of bereavement, what help might you offer?

Make some notes before reading on.

One of Sylvia's fears was that 'if I rely on others, they may let me down'. She needed encouragement to support herself and so develop confidence by doing things in her own time and in her own way. She needed reassurance that it was acceptable to resist the well-meaning demands of others. Small decisions can restore a sense of control. Major decisions need to be deferred unless they are essential, whilst the person is grieving and unable to predict what they might want to do in the future. 'I think I must be going mad!' she joked, but with an anxious look. She needed reassurance about the normality of her strong emotions and confused feelings.

Another way of viewing bereavement is as a major stress. Stress management techniques can be both useful and appropriate. Tension and anxiety can be relieved by many different approaches. A health assessment that takes into account patterns of living and personal preferences can lead to appropriate suggestions. These might include the following:

- a healthy diet;
- exercise – swimming, walking, jogging, keep fit, weight training, team sports;
- adult education classes, support groups, local interest groups;
- yoga, t'ai chi, pilates;
- relaxation, guided imagery, meditation;
- massage, aromatherapy, reflexology.

Sylvia decided to go to art classes rather than a self-help group, and booked herself a monthly massage as a treat. She began to try different audiotapes to find the type of relaxation that suited her. Reviewing progress over a period of time can be helpful, and Sylvia liked the idea of keeping a diary to record her feelings. This can be a useful tool for expressing emotions and demonstrating progress.

Box 10.10: Self-assessment question

What suggestions could you make that might help with difficult times?

Managing low points calls for some contingency plans. For many bereaved people, weekends, Sundays and bank holidays are particularly low points, with Christmas being the hardest of all. There will be other anniversaries known only to the bereaved themselves. Planning support and diversions well in advance for these times seems to help. Betty, an elderly widow who dreaded Sundays, decided to invite three other people living on their own for lunch. This was so successful that it led to a roast dinner at each other's house in turn. Her brave gesture changed the worst time to the high spot of the week for them all. Sometimes it may be possible for us to facilitate this type of support by introducing bereaved people to each other on an individual basis or via some kind of support group.

Box 10.11: Self-assessment question

What types of support are available in the locality in which you work?

Types of support are variable depending on where one lives. When working in a new area it is always necessary to find out what services and amenities are available. These include the following:

- professional counsellors may be helpful for those at risk;
- complementary therapists, who share a holistic approach and can be very valuable sources of help and support;
- the local Sport and Leisure Centre for health, fitness and recreation;
- Adult Education classes for leisure and learning;
- befriending schemes for bereaved people (e.g. home visits by supervised volunteers from the local hospice, Macmillan service, Age Concern, church groups);
- therapeutic groups which may be open or closed;
- self-help groups such as Cruse (for widows and widowers), The Compassionate Friends (for parents who have lost a child) and Gingerbread (for single parents).

Box 10.12: Key point

You might start a group yourself and facilitate it for a set period with the expressed aim of the members taking it over afterwards, if they wish to do so.

The deceptively simple skill of listening can be very powerful. Feeling that we have been fully heard can in itself be therapeutic. This can be enhanced by learning to be comfortable with silence. We can learn to convey a relaxed and unhurried approach and to resist interrupting on the assumption that we already know what is about to be said.[15] It is often our own feelings of inadequacy or embarrassment that prevent us from offering opportunities to listen and give support.

Box 10.13:   Self-assessment question

How can we care for ourselves as well as the bereaved people with whom we work?

Helping bereaved people is a special challenge. Bereavement touches us personally, reminding us of our own losses and vulnerability. Feelings of apprehension may be brought to the fore by a similar loss to that which we ourselves fear. It is painful to witness another's distress.

As we saw at the beginning of this chapter, where there is attachment followed by separation, there will be loss. As nurses, we become attached to certain patients and their families, and in some situations it may be difficult for us to let go.

Possible pitfalls include the following:

- not setting an agenda;
- inappropriate friendship;
- transference;
- counter-transference;
- negative feelings;
- being a martyr;
- not seeking support.

It is possible for bereavement support to end up as a social event rather than a helpful encounter, and so the aims and *agenda* need to be reviewed regularly. Encouragement can be very helpful, but needs to be balanced by sensitivity to the times when people are not coping and may need permission to be vulnerable. 'You are doing well!' can be a good way of stopping them telling you that the opposite is true.

It is good to feel needed, and when you – the helper – are feeling vulnerable it can be tempting to continue the relationship because you are being appreciated. There is a fine line between *friendship* and a *therapeutic relationship*. It may be useful to ask yourself whose needs you are meeting.

Ground rules for the relationship need to be set. *Transference* refers to the situation where a bereaved person transfers their feelings on to you, and you could find yourself inadvertently taking on the role of their partner, parent, child or best friend.

Self-awareness can also help you to deal with *counter-transference*. This occurs when the bereaved person reminds you of someone else. For example, you may find it difficult to be with a particular bereaved person. On reflection, you realise that this is because they remind you of someone you dislike. If you are unable to change your perception of them, then you need to refer them to someone else for help.

It is not easy to own up to *negative feelings*, yet it is impossible to be entirely non-judgemental. People's beliefs, attitudes and ways of coping may evoke strong responses in us. It is necessary to look at these uncomfortable feelings rather than deny them.

Another pitfall is to become overly concerned with our work and unwilling to let go of our relationship with a bereaved person, thinking that they may be unable to manage without us. This *martyr syndrome* leads to exhaustion in us and dependency in them.

We need to *seek support* on a regular basis. Sometimes we may not know where to find it or how to benefit from it. The longer we do not express how we feel, the more difficult it will become to do it. We need to find a safe place to share our feelings.

Regular supervision either individually or in a group can prevent this kind of build-up. If such supervision is unavailable, then it is necessary to seek this support, perhaps by pairing with another member of the team (e.g. as in co-counselling). It is important to formalise such arrangements, to adhere to time limits and to ensure that each member of the pair has an equal opportunity to speak and to listen.

Box 10.14:   Self-assessment question

What can we learn from working with bereaved people?

We are likely to find that this can be rewarding as well as challenging. Parkes and colleagues[16] point out that 'with proper training and support we shall find that repeated griefs, far from undermining our humanity and our care, enable us to cope more confidently and more sensitively with each succeeding loss'.

Working with bereaved people can teach us to value our close relationships and to give them our time and energy. We are reminded that love is a precious gift that we should appreciate while we can.

References

1   Bowlby J (1980) *Attachment and Loss. Volume 1*. Penguin, Harmondsworth.

2   Parkes CM (1998) Bereavement in adult life. *BMJ*. **316**: 856.

3   Stroebe W and Stroebe MS (eds) (1987) *Bereavement and Health*. Cambridge University Press, Cambridge.

4   Parkes CM (1964) The effects of bereavement on physical and mental health: a study of the medical records of widows. *BMJ*. **2**: 274–9.

5   Parkes CM (1998) *Bereavement: Studies of Grief in Adult Life*. Penguin, Harmondsworth.

6   Gorer G (1987) *Death, Grief and Mourning in Contemporary Britain*. Ayer Co, USA.

7   Torrie M (1975) *Begin Again: a Book for Women Alone* (2e). Dent, London.

8   Lewis CS (1991) *A Grief Observed*. Faber & Faber, London.

9   Parkes CM (1993) Bereavement as a psychosocial transition: processes of adaptation to change. In: D Dickenson and M Johnson (eds) *Death, Dying and Bereavement*. Sage Publications, London.

10   Worden WJ (1991) *Grief Counselling and Grief Therapy: A Handbook for the Mental Health Practitioner* (2e). Routledge, London.

11   Holmes TH and Rahe RH (1967) The social readjustment rating scale. *J Psychosomatic Res.* **11**: 213–18.

12   Callahan M and Kelley P (1992) *Final Gifts: Undertsanding and Helping the Dying.* Hodder & Stoughton, London.

13   Parkes CM and Weiss RS (1995) *Recovery From Bereavement.* J Aronson, USA.

14   Silverman P (1974) Anticipatory grief from the perspective of widowhood. In: Scheonberg, Carr, Kutcher *et al.* (eds) *Anticipatory Grief.* Columbia University Press, New York.

15   Burnard P (1992) *Counselling: a Guide for Practice in Nursing.* Stanley Thornes, Cheltenham.

16   Parkes CM, Relf M and Couldrick A (1996) *Counselling in Terminal Care and Bereavement.* BPS Books, London.

To learn more

Dickenson D and Johnson M (1993) *Death, Dying and Bereavement.* Sage Publications, London.

Faulkner A (1995) *Working with Bereaved People.* Churchill Livingstone, Edinburgh.

Ironside V (1996) *'You'll Get Over It': the Rage of Bereavement.* Penguin, Harmondsworth.

Parkes CM (1998) Bereavement. In: D Doyle, G Hanks and N Macdonald (eds) *Oxford Textbook of Palliative Medicine* (2e). Oxford Medical Publications, London.

Penson J (1990) *Bereavement: a Guide for Nurses.* Chapman & Hall, London.

Penson J (1995) Bereavement. In: J Penson and R Fisher (eds) *Palliative Care for People with Cancer* (2e). Edward Arnold, London.

Wallbank S (1992) *The Empty Bed.* Darton, Longman & Todd, London.

Ward B (1993) *Healing Grief: a Guide to Loss and Recovery.* Vermilion, London.

PART THREE

Working together to provide palliative care

Making the most of palliative care services
Section 1: The role of the specialist nurse

Francesca Thompson

The art and science of palliative care nursing

'It is well to give when asked, but it is better to give unasked through understanding.'[1]

Käppeli[2] suggests that the concept of nursing has a symbolic connotation. Its original language is not deemed to be precise. Interest in what constitutes the essence of nursing knowledge has developed steadily in the UK since the 1960s, stimulated by the growth in undergraduate and postgraduate education, and in nursing research.[3] Perhaps it is the ever-changing interpretation of the concept of 'nursing' which represents its essence? Käppeli[2] believes that, like any other forms of art, nursing includes three basic components, namely structure, substance, and holes to be filled with our own inspiration and imagination.

Several papers[2–8] have both supported and explored the principle that nursing practice demands the need for sound knowledge and theory. However, any theories which disregard the realities of life at the bedside are generally less attractive to nurses. A recent study[9] which examined the value that terminally ill patients place on communication and kindness shown by the community staff would endorse this view.

Davies,[4] in a review of the literature on the supportive role of the nurse in palliative care, cites several sources which suggest that care of the dying patient is essentially a nursing issue, rather than a medical one. Kennedy[3] takes this one step further and explores different ways of knowing in relation to nursing, suggesting that nurses working in this field require both 'knowing that' scientific knowledge and 'knowing how', which may be regarded as personal, experiential knowledge.

For example:[3]

Knowing that:
Pain is a complex physiological
  and emotional experience

Knowing how:
To comfort a patient who is
  distressed by severe pain

The literature[5,6,10] also describes the ability of 'expert' nurses to assess the whole picture, as well as being able to focus on relevant information. The expert nurse has the ability to sort cues, knows the right question to ask, and can respond quickly to the situation. Every person has their own story to tell in their own way and in their own time. The story may alter depending on the person to whom they are telling it, or they may not have told it before. They need to start at their own beginning.

Exercise 11.1:   Clinical mastery in getting to know the patient

Choose a person who springs to mind (a palliative care patient would be ideal, but this is not essential).

Now think back.

- What did your intuition tell you?
- What were the cues?
- Did you ignore them?
- How did their story unfold?
- Did you facilitate this?
- How did you synthesise the information?
- Did you record it?
- How did you feel at the time?
- How do you feel now?
- What did you learn about the person?
- What did you learn about yourself?
- Would you do things differently with hindsight?

The nurse specialist debate
Role boundaries

More than any other group, nurses have close daily contact with patients. Nursing services account for approximately 25% of the total NHS budget, and 80% of direct care is delivered by nurses.[11]

The Primary Healthcare Team is central to the provision of palliative care, reinforced by recent Government strategic policies.[12,13] Most of the last year of life is spent at home,[14] with a significant number of cancer patients and their families hoping to fulfil their desire to die at home.[15] Because of this, the nurse is required to respond rapidly to ongoing scientific and medical technological advances, complex economic factors and changes in the patterns of care. This in itself heralds exciting entrepreneurial and leadership opportunities for nursing, rather than a temptation to defend functions and roles that are obsolete.

The specific role of the 'specialist' community nurse emerges as that of practising with a working knowledge of the community, the residents, the organisation and distribution of healthcare services, the population and the network of other care providers.[16] Certainly there has been a dramatic increase in both medical and nursing specialisation, which should aim to complement this existing primary generalist expertise. It is only the speciality of the intervention that is different.

In palliative care the task that lies ahead is often complex and open to interpretation. The goal is to improve the *quality of life* for both the patient and their family.

- What does this mean?
- What needs to be done?
- Who is best equipped to assist in the task?
- Who would the patient prefer to be helped by?
- What is any given individual's role in working towards the task?

Several sources[9,17–20] highlight the need to address roles and responsibilities within palliative care. Lack of clarity results in themes of inter- and intra-conflict, disempowerment and burnout.[17]

Role definition

Castledine[21] has explored the varying perspectives on nursing practice in the UK. Whatever the view, this debate draws parallel to recent proliferation of the number and types of specialist nursing posts. For example, Bowman and Thompson,[22] consider that the current problem with 'nurse specialists' is that they develop in a system which organises patients into groups that are convenient for medical strategies. Undoubtedly, the process of specialisation in nursing practice aims for an improvement in patient care, but when providing cancer nursing services it is important to differentiate between a nurse working in a speciality and a specialist nurse.[11]

Bousfield's[17] findings suggest that clinical nurse specialists are experienced practitioners who strive to occupy positions where they can influence patient care and utilize advanced knowledge, expertise and leadership skills in a multidisciplinary environment.

The literature[10,11,17,21] further proposes that, for the role of the clinical nurse specialist to be recognised and accepted, individuals need to be educated at an advanced level, demonstrate practice based in research, and have a firm base as specialists in nursing.

The Post-Registration Education and Practice (PREP)[23] report recognised the limitations of current pre-registration nurse education in the UK in meeting the needs of professional practice which is focused on the delivery of specialist care and case management in the community.

The United Kingdom Central Council for Nursing, Midwifery and Health Visiting (UKCC)[23] now defines a specialist nursing practitioner as someone:

> *'able to demonstrate higher levels of clinical decision-making. Able to monitor and improve standards of care through supervision of practice, clinical audit, the provision of skilled professional leadership and the development of practice through research, teaching and the support of professional colleagues.'*

In December 1997, the UKCC agreed that further clarification and development work should be undertaken in this area.[24] Subsequent research has highlighted the need for a clear and robust framework across the UK to recognise a standard for a higher level of practice. Their perspective is such that not every practitioner will become a specialist practitioner. In fact, there will always be only a minority of the profession working at this higher level. However, the point at issue is how to regulate this level of practice for the safety of the public and, as such, a recent update[25] shows overwhelming support for a move by the UKCC towards recognising nurses, midwives and health visitors who are working at this level.

Role transition

The Calman/Hine report[12] highlights the importance of creating a network of care which will enable a patient, wherever he or she lives, to be sure that the treatment is of a uniformly high standard. The Royal College of Nursing (RCN)[26] believes that for this to happen, patients affected by cancer must have access to nurses with the appropriate experience and skills. However, it is important to note that although there has been an increasing emphasis on post-registration qualification for specialist practice,[11,27] there are other areas of equal value in responding to the following question (*see* Exercise 11.2).

Finally, if you are considering working towards a clinical nurse specialist (CNS) post, or you are newly appointed, it is worthwhile planning for the transition[29–31] and analysing your role through the next exercise (*see* Exercise 11.3).

Referral, intervention and outcome

The clinical nurse specialist (CNS) role is based on enabling and empowering others. The reason for referral to a specialist service will therefore be to seek either participa-

---

Exercise 11.2:   How can I become a clinical nurse specialist (CNS) in palliative care? (Adapted[28])

- *Have I got what it takes to be a CNS?*

Apart from a deep commitment to and interest in palliative care, clinical nurse specialists should be prepared to become involved in the indirect aspects of care, such as teaching, research, and strategy- and policy-making. Confidence and leadership skills are essential as many posts, although part of a team, may demand working in isolation or autonomously.

- *What kind of experience do I need?*

Five years of post-registration experience, with at least a recent 2 years in cancer or palliative care. The role encompasses not only clinical expertise, but also consultative, teaching, leadership and research functions. Evidence of experience in teaching and advanced communication skills is essential.

- *What qualifications do I need?*

It is paramount to be clinically credible in palliative care nursing. This means taking opportunities to study for relevant courses as well as keeping up to date with the literature and/or publishing your own material. While an established CNS may not hold degrees, it is unlikely that less experienced nurses will be able to move into such posts without a willingness to work towards a first degree.

- *What grade can I expect?*

The role and responsibilities expected of a CNS demand a grade no lower than G or its equivalent.

---

tion or collaboration towards improving care for that patient and their family. In order to reach the maximum number of patients, the CNS will work within a defined framework for accepting referrals. The CNS is trained to assess situations in which the addition of their emotionlly and/or physically focused intervention *will aim to make a difference.* It is likely that the focus of care will be problem- and/or need-orientated, rather than being directed towards symptoms and treatment.

Prior to any referral, it is essential to explore the patient's experience to date, and not to underestimate their own judgement of their state of health. What we do know[32] is that a patient's previous experience of the disclosure of diagnosis and disease progression will impact upon both their information needs and their attitude towards involvement in decision-making. Consequently, careful thought about the timing of referral, and the sharing of the reasons behind it, are essential for maintaining the patient's trust and integrity.

Evidence is becoming available to demonstrate that community-based specialist palliative care is beneficial in terms of improved patient and carer satisfaction.[33]

Exercise 11.3: Role of CNS in palliative care (an example for breaking bad news)

Role components/ activities (example in clinical practice)	Time spent (%)	Underlying key skills/ knowledge needed to be successful at this level	Included in job description	Planned activity	Needs of	Emerging development need
• Breaking bad news and dealing with distress	High	• Experience in various settings • Advanced communication skills/ qualification	Yes	Yes and no	Patients and carers	• Dealing with children • Appropriate model of clinical supervision • Time-management skills
• Teaching of the above	Low	• Theory of breaking bad news • Teaching methods • Evaluating teaching/ demonstrating change in practice	Yes	Yes	Management	• Improve links with training department and post-graduate centre • Increase confidence in formal teaching of small groups
• Producing guidelines for breaking bad news	None to date	• Sharing of good practice from other areas • Clinical audit/outcome measures	Added to revised job description	Yes	Clinical governance issue	• Seek advice on forming a steering group • Plan meeting with audit department • Read the NHS White Paper (1997)

However, we also know how much value patients place on their relationship with health professionals, and on continuity of care.[9] Therefore, before introducing a specialist service, it is essential to consider what more *you* can do first. Once considered, this should elicit robust reasons from both your own and the patient's perspectives. Work through Exercise 11.4 as one way of determining your level of skill.

Exercise 11.4:   Case study

Bill has difficulty in swallowing and eating. He has rapidly advancing cancer of the oesophagus and is very frightened, particularly as he has breathing problems.

1 Can you determine the possible reasons for his breathing distress?
2 Can you list the interventions/treatment options available to him?
3 Should pleural effusions always be tapped?
4 How do you prepare patients who are likely to experience breathlessness?

Useful guidelines[34] have assisted Macmillan nurses in analysing and recording their level of intervention. Such intervention may range from straightforward telephone advice, through to holding a caseload of the more complex situations. Interestingly, Clark[35] notes the impact of social deprivation on workload. In addition to this, we have yet to see the implications for nursing practice through the Crown Report[36] and the introduction of nurse prescribing.

In conclusion, there is evidence, that improved co-ordination of local palliative care services can lead to substantial cost savings through reduced hospital admissions and the need for fewer home visits.[37] Equally, an out-of-hours study, demonstrated the merits worth of 'round-the-clock' specialist advice.[38] The investment in palliative care has created a valuable resource, but the challenge facing us now is how to use this in such a way that all patients, including those with non-cancer diagnoses, can benefit from access to improved care.

References

1   Gibran K (1991) *The Prophet*. Pan Books, London.

2   Käppeli S (1993) Advanced clinical practice – how do we promote it? *J Clin Nursing*. **2**: 205–10.

3   Kennedy C (1998) Ways of knowing in palliative nursing. *Int J Palliative Nursing*. **4**: 240–45.

4   Davies B and Oberle K (1990) Dimensions of the supportive role of the nurse in palliative care. *Oncol Nursing Forum*. **17**: 87–94.

5   Benner P, Tanner C and Chelsby C (1992) From beginner to expert: gaining a differential clinical world in critical nursing care. *Adv Nursing Sci*. **14**: 13–18.

6   Gatley P (1992) From novice to expert: the use of intuitive knowledge as a basis for district nurse education. *Nurse Education Today.* **12**: 81–7.

7   Corner J (1996) *Proceedings of the Robert Tiffany Lecture: Beyond Survival Rates and Side-Effects – Cancer Nursing as Therapy.* Ninth International Conference on Cancer Nursing, Sussex.

8   Lorensen M, Jones DE and Hamilton GA (1998) Advanced nursing practice in the Nordic countries. *J Clin Nursing.* **7**, 257–264.

9   Grande GE, Todd CJ, Barclay SIG *et al.* (1996) What terminally ill patients value in the support provided by GPs, district and Macmillan nurses. *Int J Palliative Nursing.* **2**: 138–43.

10 Kai-Cheung Chuk P (1997) Clinical nurse specialists and quality patient care. *J Adv Nursing.* **26**: 501–6.

11 RCN Cancer Nursing Society (1996) *A Structure for Cancer Nursing Services.* RCN Cancer Nursing Society, London.

12 Calman K and Hine D (1995) A policy framework for commissioning cancer services: a Report by the Expert Advisory Group on Cancer to the Chief Medical Officers of England and Wales. Department of Health and Welsh Office, London and Cardiff.

13 Department of Health (1997) *The New NHS: Modern, Dependable.* HMSO, London.

14 Cartwright A (1991) Changes in life and care in the year before death 1969–1987. *J Public Health Med.* **13**: 81–7.

15 Dunlop R, Davies RJ and Mockley JM (1989) Preferred versus actual place of death: a hospital palliative care support team experience. *Palliative Med.* **3**: 197–201.

16 Kelly A (1996) The concept of the specialist community nurse. *J Adv Nursing.* **24**: 42–52.

17 Bousfield C (1997) A phenomenological investigation into the role of the clinical nurse specialist. *J Adv Nursing.* **25**: 245–56.

18 Mystakidou K (1997) Team dynamics and the difficult patient. In: *Proceedings of the Fifth Congress of the European Association for Palliative Care*, Barcelona.

19 Hanks G (1995) The interdisciplinary team. In: D Doyle, G Hanks and N Mcdonald (eds) *Oxford Textbook of Palliative Medicine.* Oxford Medical Publications, Oxford.

20 Hill A (1998) Multiprofessional teamwork in hospital palliative care teams. *Int J Palliative Med.* **4**: 214–21.

21 Castledine G (1995) Editorial: defining specialist nursing. *Br J Nursing.* **4**: 264–5.

22 Bowman G and Thompson P (1990) When is a specialist not a specialist? *Nursing Times.* **88**: 48.

23 UKCC (1994) *PREP: the Future of Professional Practice – the Council's Standards for Education and Practice Following Registration.* UKCC, London.

24 UKCC (1997) *PREP – Specialist Practice: Consideration of Issues Relating to Embracing Nurse Practitioners and Clinical Nurse Specialists Within the Specialist Framework.* UKCC, London.

25   UKCC (1999) *Towards a Higher Level of Practice*. UKCC, London.

26   Cancer Collaboration (1997) *The Workforce and Training Implications of the Calman/Hine Cancer Report*. Research Campaign and Macmillan Cancer Relief, London.

27   RCN Cancer Nursing Society (1996) *Guidelines for Good Practice in Cancer Nursing Education*. RCN Cancer Nursing Society, London.

28   Willis J (1998) The clinical nurse specialist. *Nursing Times Learning Curve*. **2**: 14–15.

29   Glenn S and Waddington K (1998) Transition from staff nurse to clinical nurse specialist: a case study. *J Clin Nursing*. **7**: 283–90.

30   Woods LP (1998) Implementing advanced practice: identifying the factors that facilitate and inhibit the process. *J Clin Nursing*. **7**: 265–73.

31   Colquhoun M and Dougan H (1997) Performance standards: ensuring that the specialist nurse in palliative care is special. *Palliative Med*. **11**: 381–7.

32   Cawley N (1997) The experiences of patients with advanced cancer undergoing a referral to palliative care: a phenomenological study. Summary Report Prepared for Macmillan Cancer Relief, London.

33   Salisbury C, Bosanquet N, Wilkinson EK *et al.* (1999) The impact of different models of specialist palliative care on patient's quality of life: a systematic literature review. *Palliative Med*. **13**: 3–17.

34   Webber J (1993) *The Evolving Role of the Macmillan Nurse*. Macmillan Cancer Relief, London.

35   Clark CR (1997) Social deprivation increases workload in palliative care of terminally ill patients. *BMJ Letters*. **314**: 1202.

36   Department of Health (1999) *The Report of the Advisory Group on Nurse Prescribing (The Crown Report)*. HMSO, London.

37   Bosanquet N (1997) New challenge for palliative care. *BMJ*. **314**: 1294.

38   Hatcliffe S and Smith P (1997) Open all hours. *Health Service J*. **Jun**: 40–41.

39   Meystre CJN, Burley NMJ and Ahmedzai S (1997) What investigations and procedures do patients in hospices want? Interview-based survey of patients and their nurses. *BMJ*. **315**: 1202–3.

To learn more

Humphris D (1994) *The Clinical Nurse Specialist*. Macmillan Press, London.

Exercise 11.4:   Answers

1 Airflow obstruction:
   - large airways – tumour, stricture, tracheal compression;
   - small airways - asthma, chronic obstructive airways disease, lymphangitis carcinomatosa.

   Decreased lung volume – lung secondaries, extensive tumour, effusion, ascites, infection, lung collapse, pneumothorax.

   Neuromuscular failure – phrenic nerve palsy, cachexia.

   Pain – fractures, nerve/bone infiltration, pleurisy, infection.

   Decreased gas exchange – pulmonary embolism, pulmonary oedema.

   Anaemia.

   Anxiety-related causes.

2 Remove the cause if possible (i.e. treat infection, effusion, wheeze, cardiac failure).

   Treat the cause if possible (i.e. radiotherapy, steroids).

   Treat the symptom (i.e. opioids, benzodiazepines). Consider the various drug administration routes available, and identify the most appropriate one.

   Relieve the distress by listening to and emotionally supporting the patient. Reposition the patient, change bedclothes and pillows, use a bedside table or chair, use cooling fans, use breathing retraining techniques and strategies to help to overcome functional difficulties.

3 The answer is no, but there is evidence to suggest that even patients who are terminally ill are prepared to accept invasive procedures and treatments more readily than are their nurses.[39]

4 Breathlessness can be very distressing for the patient, especially if they do not know what is happening. There is evidence that if the intervention is made early enough, nurses can help patients to redefine breathlessness as a problem that they can learn to manage themselves.[7] To do this they need help to work through their fears and the limitations that these impose.

Section 2: The role of the hospice in-patient unit

Suzanne Lesley Cockerton

Introduction

Hospice care has the explicit aim of treating the family as the unit of care. Strong emphasis is placed on patient autonomy and, where indicated by the patient, disclosure of the prognosis, the ultimate aim being to allow informed choices about care and treatment. The focus of this care lies in the following:

- supporting informal carers through a time of stress and bereavement;
- maintaining their involvement with the care of the patient;
- bringing the comfort of home into what would otherwise be institutional care.

The hospice philosophy stresses the importance of an individual approach to caring. This is achieved by multiprofessional and inter-agency working within a non-hierarchical environment with favourable staffing levels.[1]

Referral

It is acknowledged that most of the final year of life is spent at home and that care is provided by relatives. Therefore the responsibility falls to the primary care team to inform and refer to in-patient services.[2]

Access to in-patient services may come from any source, including the following:

- hospitals;
- social services;
- non-statutory agencies.

Referral is subject to the general practitioner agreeing to specialist involvement with the patient.[3] It is vital that the providers of in-patient services are clear about their service provision and that it is supported by a written policy statement. This admission policy must be readily available for professionals and agencies to view. The content should cover the criteria for acceptance and reinforce the intent of the hospice to support and complement the care provided by primary healthcare teams, statutory and non-statutory agencies and hospitals. This will assist healthcare professionals in selecting the appropriate patients for referral to the hospice service.

In-patient units are managed so as to provide specific palliative care interventions. They are not long-stay units, and a typical length of stay would be 7–14 days (see Boxes 11.1 and 11.2 for suggested admission criteria).

Box 11.1:   Criteria for admission to the in-patient unit

1 Admissions to the in-patient unit should be planned, where possible with a minimum of 24 hours' notice.
2 Reasons for admission will usually be as follows.
3 3.1 Symptom control.
   3.2 Terminal care (i.e. death likely within 5–7 days).
   3.3 Assessment or reassessment of physical, psychosocial and spiritual needs.
   3.4 Specific interventions (e.g. blood transfusion, paracentesis and chest drainage).
   3.5 Respite care (see Box 11.2 for respite criteria).
4 Acceptance of a patient for admission will take into account the availability of a bed and the multidisciplinary team resources.
5 Patients will not usually be accepted if they suffer from a psychotic illness coexistent with the physical condition for which they are seeking treatment, unless the psychiatrist caring for them confirms that their mental state is not a danger to themselves or to others.
6 The Medical Director has principal responsibility for the admission and discharge of the patients, working closely with the nursing staff of the in-patient unit and day hospice and other members of the multidisciplinary team.
7 Before a decision is made to transfer a patient from the local hospitals, the Medical Director or hospital Macmillan nurse will visit the patient to assist in the preparation of the patient and family and to ensure that the move to the hospice is appropriate for all concerned.

Box 11.2:   Respite philosophy

1 The hospice recognises the need for respite care for patients/families with palliative care needs. It aims to provide a flexible, responsive service to the community. Respite care will be seen as a palliative intervention.
2 Respite can be requested for all patients with palliative care needs, whatever their

diagnosis, unless the hospice is an unsuitable environment for their care (e.g. those with serious mental health problems or dementia).

3 All patients/families requesting respite care will have their needs assessed in the community by a member of the multidisciplinary team.

4 The frequency and duration of the respite stays will depend upon need, and assessments will be an ongoing process. Stays will normally be for a 7-day period.

5 Patients without palliative care needs will be offered advice and information about alternative services.

6 In cases where a patient who did not previously have palliative care needs, but has by the progressive nature of their illness developed these, reassessment of need will be undertaken.

7 Requests for crisis respite care must be discussed on a doctor-to-doctor basis and in consultation with the clinical manager for the in-patient and day hospice services.

Collaboration and team work

In-patient units are in a position to emulate collaboration and teamwork which can lead to excellent care. This is achieved by establishing a team of individuals who:

- agree on the prime task of delivering a high standard of patient-led care;
- have a commitment to improve what is done and how it is done;
- will make decisions and ensure the implementation of these;
- communicate openly;
- are generous and offer mutual support for all members;
- participate and listen to each other;
- allow disagreement and do not allow conflict to be personalised;
- know that they belong and have a sense of loyalty to the work group.

Collaboration simply means working together. Inter-professional collaboration is the willingness to share and give up exclusive claims to specialised knowledge and authority if the needs of the patient can be met more efficiently by other professions.[4] Individual professionals will often have a limited view of the patient's situation. Therefore the care of the dying must involve a team approach to ensure that the complexities of the problems and the needs presented are addressed.

The nature of teamwork has been subject to much exploration.[5] Effective teamwork within in-patient settings is based on the following:

- shared goals and objectives which take into account the values of individual staff;
- complementary roles which are understood and respected by team members;
- clear procedures and agreed guidelines for practice;
- regular and effective communication;
- support and recognition of each member's role;
- regular audit and reflection on practice.

A fundamental element of building an effective team is leadership. Leaders of in-patient services need to balance the ability to involve all members of the team in a process of democratic decision-making with the ability to resolve differences, forge a sense of purpose and provide guidance.[6]

Model of in-patient care

The key to first-rate in-patient care which encompasses the physical, psychosocial and spiritual dimensions lies in *attention to detail*. This requires a pro-active approach in order to search for and identify the problems and needs of the patient and their family. Although relief of physical distress remains the first priority, it should not be allowed to become the ultimate goal. The alleviation of physical symptoms is just the beginning of what can be offered to patients and their families. Dying is not simply a biological fact, but an experience that is grounded in the social relationships that have been established between the patient, their family and the society in which they live.[7] This psychosocial perspective of care is concerned with the psychological and emotional well-being of the patient and their family. It helps to enlighten the meaning of dying and the resulting behaviour of the patient.[8,9] In-patient care can provide an environment that fosters therapeutic relationships in order to establish a greater depth of understanding between the professional and the patient. Once established, it is the tool that will enable the multidisciplinary team to apply humanistic principles of care[*] in order to meet individual needs.

The challenge for in-patient teams is to respond appropriately to the physical symptoms of the dying process while not allowing the medical aspects of the patient's situation to obscure the profoundly personal nature of the experience for the individual. The dying process includes the physical, psychological and spiritual deterioration that the patient will experience.

Support for families is an important dimension of the total hospice caring approach. Relatives are under great stress during a family member's terminal illness, and the in-patient team have the skills that are needed to provide sensitive support.

The philosophy of in-patient care should be aimed at reducing patient and family anxiety and their sense of losing control. Support needs to be directed as far as possible to enabling people to manage their own lives, rather than taking that responsibility away from them.[10] Promoting self-care and facilitating the individual's performance can contribute to that person's sense of well-being.

Inadequate communication can cause more problems than any other factor in terminal care. The personal one-to-one relationships between patients, relatives and specialist nurses are difficult to replicate in the in-patient setting. However, many units have adapted a form of primary nursing or a key-worker role. A primary nurse

---

[*]This requires the professional to understand the human nature of the patient and to possess a belief in human effort, rather than in religion.

or key-worker model requires the allocation of a named nurse or other professional to the patient. This primary nurse or key-worker has responsibility for co-ordinating the care of their allocated patient in collaboration with the multidisciplinary team. The role will also provide a focal point for all communication about the patient. This ensures that an allocated nurse or other professional maintains responsibility for assessing, planning and evaluating patient care and providing the family with support.[10]

Specialist professionals within in-patient services

Many professionals work within the in-patient unit in order to help patients to achieve an optimum quality of life.

These areas of expertise include the following.

- Complimentary therapies provide additional attention, hope, comfort and care for patients. The therapies most frequently offered are aromatherapy, massage and stress-reduction techniques.
- Creative and diversional activities are of benefit to patients in that they can increase independence and a sense of self-worth and purpose.
- Physiotherapy provides assessment of physical ability to promote mobility and independence.
- Lymphoedema treatment can provide comfort and improve function in the affected area.
- Occupational therapy can provide therapeutic interventions (e.g. energy conservation) and address specific problems associated with discharge planning.
- Speech therapy can suggest measures to restore speech and aid the patient's ability to swallow.
- Chiropody can help to reduce or remove discomfort and maintain mobility.
- Dietitians provide advice on the maintenance of a realistic food intake.
- Chaplaincy staff provide specific religious ministry as well as generalised pastoral/ spiritual care.
- Family support teams provide emotional support with specific expertise in family therapy and working with bereaved children and adolescents. Advice about benefits and financial assistance is also provided.
- Bereavement services provide a combination of professional and volunteer bereavement support in the form of visiting or befriending, support groups and specialist bereavement counselling.
- Counselling provides specific, specialised counselling involving the setting of boundaries of time and place, using the British Association of Counselling guidelines.
- Nurses have the expertise to give practical nursing care and to teach the patient to self-care. Nursing input is extended by communicating and supplying information which can help to optimise the patient's lifestyle.

- Medical input for the patient is provided according to the stage of the disease. It may be active, supportive or palliative, diagnosing and treating symptoms of continuing disease as they arise. There are situations where the stress of the disease will result in mental health disorders including anxiety and depression.
- Referral to a psychiatrist or counsellor may be indicated. The treatment offered may include counselling, psychological intervention (including cognitive behavioural therapy) and drug treatment.

Evaluation and audit

Improving the quality of palliative care is the goal of most professionals. Audit can help in-patient services in the following ways.

- Staff are able to monitor and review the quality of their work and seek ways to improve it.
- Audit provides a systematic way of thinking about objectives and outcomes of care.
- Audit identifies areas where care is effective and where it is not.

Typical examples of audit tools used in palliative care settings are the Edmonton Symptom Assessment System (ESAS) and the Support Team Assessment Schedule (STAS).[11]

Conclusion

When a patient is admitted to an in-patient unit, they are in danger of becoming a passive recipient of care, with nurses doing too much for them and therefore teaching them to become passive and helpless. The family is likely to be displaced as they hand over the responsibility of care to the professionals. If the varied needs of both the patient and their family are to be met, a multiprofessional team approach is required. The development of a confiding relationship between the patient, their family and members of the team is an important aspect of the care that is given. It is of primary importance that the patient trusts the professional providing the care and support. The success of hospice in-patient care is apparent when the patient and their family are enabled to resume responsibility for the patient's care if this is their wish, by being involved and allowed to continue with personal care tasks.

A sense of purpose for the patient and their family is also achieved when they actively participate in the communication process and are fully informed of the patient's situation. In circumstances where the patient and family are unable, unwilling or refuse to take back the carer role, the multiprofessional team can continue to give the care that is required with commitment, having sufficient skills to uphold the integrity of both the patient and their family.

Chapter 11, Section 2:   Questions

1 What is meant by a 'whole-person' approach to patient care?
2 What are the benefits of a primary nurse/key-worker role?
3 Who maintains the principal responsibility for patient care whilst in the community?
4 What are the reasons for admission to a hospice in-patient unit?
5 What is meant by becoming a 'passive recipient of care'?

References

1   Neale B (1991) *Informal Palliative Care. A Review of Research on Needs, Standards and Service Evaluation*. Occasional Paper No. 3. Trent Palliative Care Centre.

2   Department of Health (1992) *The Principles and Provision of Palliative Care. Joint Report of the Standing Medical Advisory Committee and Standing Nursing and Midwifery Advisory Committee*. HMSO, London.

3   Doyle D (1997) *Dilemmas and Directions: the Future of Specialist Palliative Care*. Occasional Paper No. 11. National Council for Hospice and Specialist Palliative Care Services, London.

4   Scott G (1995) Challenging conventional roles in palliative care. *Nursing Times*. **91**: 3.

5   Harwood A (1997) Leadership: spot the saboteurs. *Nursing Times*. **93**: 73–4.

6   McSherry R and Browne J (1997) Leader's tools of the trade. *Nursing Times*. **93**: 70–2.

7   Radley A (1994) *Making Sense of Illness: the Social Psychology of Health and Illness*. Sage Publications, London.

8   Byock I (1996) Beyond symptom management. *Eur J Palliative Care*. **3**: 125–30.

9   National Council for Hospice and Specialist Palliative Care Services (1997) *Feeling Better: Psychosocial Care in Specialist Palliative Care. A Discussion Paper*. Occasional Paper No. 13. London National Council.

10   Bliss J and Johnson B (1995) After diagnosis of cancer: the patient's view of life. *Int J Palliative Nursing*. **1**: 126–33.

11   Higginson I (ed) (1993) *Clinical Audit in Palliative Care*. Radcliffe Medical Press, Oxford.

To learn more

Goldberg R and Tull R (1983) *The Psychosocial Dimension of Cancer: A Practical Guide for Health Care Providers*. The Free Press, New York.

Oliviere D, Hargreave R and Monroe B (1997) *Good Practice in Palliative Care*. Ashgate Publishing, Aldershot.

Tschudin V (1995) *Nursing the Patient with Cancer*. Prentice-Hall, Hemel Hempstead.

Chapter 11, Section 2:   Answers

1 This requires the professional to understand the human nature of the patient and to possess a belief in human effort, rather than in religion.
2 The benefits of the primary nurse or key-worker role are as follows.

- An individual professional takes responsibility for co-ordinating the care given to the patient and their family by the multidisciplinary team.
- An individual professional takes responsibility for assessing, planning and evaluating patient care.
- An individual professional provides a focal point for all communication about the patient.

3 The patient's general practitioner.
4 The reasons for admission to a hospice in-patient unit are as follows:

- symptom control;
- terminal care (i.e. in cases where death is likely within 5–7 days);
- assessment or reassessment of physical, psychosocial and spiritual needs;
- specific interventions (e.g. blood transfusion, paracentesis and chest drainage);
- respite care.

5 This occurs when professionals do too much for the patient and their family, thereby minimising their resources and abilities. This leads to a reduced likelihood of maintaining and promoting patient and family independence.

Section 3: The role of the hospice day unit

Pearl McDaid

Introduction

Hospice or palliative day care was piloted in the mid 1970s, and is now established as an important component of care for those suffering from progressive and life-limiting illnesses. There are at present 251 hospice day-care centres listed in the *1999 Directory of Hospice Services in the UK and Republic of Ireland* compiled by the Hospice Information Service at St Christopher's Hospice, London.

Hospice day care is complementary to all other cancer services, and provides support for and surveillance of patients which could not otherwise be achieved either in hospital or in the community. The primary aims of this form of care are therefore to assist in the enhancement of the *quality of life* of these patients by means of liaison and effective communication with all concerned.[1]

Accessing day care

Who can refer?

Local hospice or palliative care service policies will govern the route of access when referring a patient to day care, but generally the needs of the patient and family carers are identified by a healthcare professional from the hospice, hospital or community settings (*see* Figure 11.1).

In many instances the referral is made by a healthcare professional directly to the day-care service, and it is often preceded by a telephone call. In other cases, it is policy for the referral to be made through the Macmillan Nursing Service or Hospice Home Care Nursing Service.

Information about the referral policy can be obtained from the local hospice or palliative care service.

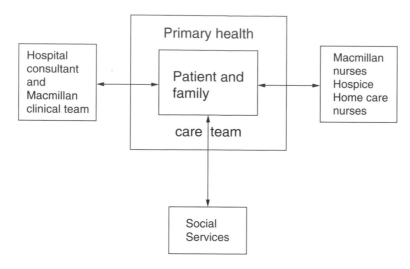

Figure 11.1   Routes of access when referring a patient to day care.

How to refer

It is usual for a *referral form* to be completed giving as much relevant information as possible (and as space allows), together with clear and objective reasons for referral. It may also be helpful if the referrer includes copies of summary letters relating to the patient's condition.

If a *referral letter* is the required method of referral, the same relevant information, and clear and objective reasons for referral should be included.

If in doubt, contact the Hospice Day-Care Unit by telephone for advice!

Why refer, and when?

For many patients, the diagnosis and treatment of malignant disease is a major intrusion into their lives and the lives of their families. In the short term, the focus is on treatment options and coming to terms with the knowledge of their illness. Despite the plethora of articles and information which have been published in newspapers and magazines, many people retain pre-existing fears and phobias regarding cancer and cancer treatments. Dealing with these problems at this stage, is within the domain of the Macmillan or clinical nurse or doctor specialists. Long-term plans for the patient remain uncertain.

For those patients whose disease is life-threatening, many adjustments will have to be made to their lifestyles. They are often too incapacitated to resume their usual roles, routines and hobbies. Quite often they and their families are left stunned by the situation. Many are still recovering from the effects of anti-cancer treatments, and it is often at this stage that the Community Nursing Service becomes more actively involved in the patient's care, together with the general practitioner or other members of the Primary Healthcare team (PHCT).

It may well be that a member of the PHCT notices that the patient's mood is low, and that they have lost the confidence to resume activities that are well within their physical capabilities. Their mood is variable – often they feel sad rather than depressed, and they appear unable to motivate themselves, although they are reluctantly motivated by others. They are often all too aware of the strain this puts on their family carers, and they feel both responsible and guilty. A patient who cannot return to work in the foreseeable future (if ever), or who previously normally had an active social life, will be trying to adjust to the change of lifestyle brought about by their illness.

Physical symptoms may be difficult to manage because they may be exacerbated by anxiety or worry. Sleep patterns may be fragmented and dysfunctional, and the patient's appetite may be poor.

It is for those patients who are not actually dying, but whose ability to fulfil their usual roles is compromised – both within their families and in society – that referral to hospice day care is indicated.

Summary of criteria for referral

1 *The patient who is physically isolated or incapacitated due to illness or treatments*: may benefit from advice and treatment for physical symptoms, and help with activities of daily living from day-care professionals.
2 *The patient who is emotionally isolated due to illness or treatments*: may benefit from peer group support and companionship, counselling, diversion or complementary therapies.
3 *The patient who is experiencing difficulty in adjusting to changes in role, status or function within their family or in society*: may benefit from counselling from day-care professionals, and peer group support.
4 *The family that is experiencing stress due to the patient's illness, and changes in their roles, status and function*: may benefit from advice or counselling from a social worker, and the respite which hospice day care offers.
5 *Anticipation that future advice and support will be needed by the PHCT to*:
   • manage the patient's care and symptom control at home;
   • cope with family issues or bereavement.

Criteria for admission to day unit

There is generally a written policy regarding the criteria for admission to the hospice day-care service, which identifies those patients for whom the service is provided, and a broad outline of the range (and limitations) of facilities that are available. It is likely that an initial assessment has already been made either by the day-care leader visiting the patient and their family at home, or when the patient and a family member visited the day unit to look round. However, the policy in many organisations is for a formal assessment of the patient's and family's needs to take place prior to admission to day care.

Assessment

Although formal, the assessment should be open and relaxed, and is focused on the patient as a person, and the effect that the disease and treatments have had on them, their family and their lifestyles.

Russell[2] uses the following format for assessment of the patient:

- review of the illness, and the patient's perception and understanding of it;
- current problems, including a review of medication;
- physical abilities and limitations;
- social situation and the level of support available for the patient and their family;
- mood and morale;
- insight, including the patient's ideas, concerns and expectations;
- clinical examination (as appropriate).

At the conclusion of the assessment, the problems should be prioritised and recorded, and the outcome of the consultation should be discussed with the patient and their family carer, including their suitability for day care. Some patients need to be admitted to day care for a limited period only if care objectives can be achieved and they become well and confident enough to cope. However, for the majority of cases this is not feasible. An appointment should be made for a *review assessment*, which evaluates the care given and received, and further care objectives should be set, together with another review date.

Normally, patients attend day care for one day a week, and the most suitable day needs to be negotiated and transport requirements ascertained and organised. A letter summarising the assessment should be sent to the patient's GP, and copies sent to other relevant professionals.

What is hospice or palliative day care and what does it offer?

In 1998, a telephone survey of the provision of palliative day-care services was published[3] which collected data in order to identify the nature of palliative day-care provision in the UK. The results provided information on the following:

- the nature of the service;
- the range and types of service;
- management and organisational issues;
- common care problems and care issues for patients attending day care.

This survey[3] found that hospice and palliative day-care units operate for between one and six days a week to provide a service for mainly adult cancer patients (97%) and patients with other progressive life-limiting diseases (e.g. motor neurone disease or HIV/AIDs).

The model of care ranges from the medical model (with its strong emphasis on medical input) to the social model (with its emphasis on social activities), and is influenced by the locality of the day unit and the needs of the community which it serves. However, *medical input* is provided for the majority of day units, and all of them employ at least one *Registered General Nurse*.

Day care provides the following:

- regular monitoring and surveillance of symptom control;
- access to a specialist multiprofessional team;
- mutual respite for both patient and carer;
- psychosocial support;
- peer group support.

Day care aims to provide a service that enables the patient to make adjustments in physical and psychological terms, in order to achieve his or her full potential in the circumstances. Initially, for some new patients, advice and help with physical problems are priorities, while for others the priority is a desperate need to talk about their concerns and anxieties to a professional. Often solace is found in observing and talking to other patients who have had similar experiences, and who have accepted their situation, adjusted their lifestyle and are coping. Thus feelings of belonging and safety are engendered, and the patient's self-esteem and confidence begin to emerge to the point where they are able to express their opinions and initiate comment and discussion.

Staffing and services provided

The demands of the service will determine the size and skill mix of the team. Volunteers' skills are widely utilised in day care to support the staff in a variety of ways, ranging from driving patients to and from the day unit and hostess duties, to professionally trained people offering their services voluntarily.

All day units employ or have access to registered nurses who provide nursing care and advice, and who liaise with other professional specialists and their community colleagues about the patients' well-being. Healthcare assistants may also form part of the team providing supervised nursing care.

Many day units have facilities for hair dressing and manicuring.

Complementary therapies are now commonly used adjuvants for relaxation, to promote a feeling of well-being and maximise control of pain and symptoms.

Aromatherapy consists of massage with essential oils for relaxation, relief of aches and pains or stiffness of a joint, and to promote a feeling of well-being. Each oil has its own individual therapeutic properties and the therapist chooses the oil(s) which are most appropriate for the patient's needs.

The following therapies are based on the Far Eastern belief that the body's health and well-being are dependent on the free flow of energy through the meridians or pathways that are situated throughout the body. Obstruction of or interference with this energy flow is thought to be the cause of physical disorders.

Acupuncture is the introduction of very fine needles into the skin over relevant points of the body in order to release and promote the flow of energy.

Reflexology follows the same principles of the flow of energy through the meridians, but according to this therapy each organ and part of the body has a corresponding zone in the feet, and therefore pressure is applied to that zone by the therapist.

Shiatsu massage frees the flow of energy through the meridians by massage.

Reiki healing is 'hands on' healing in which the healer channels the external universal life-force energy through their own hands of the healer to the patient's body.

Creative and diversional activities feature widely in day care, and include painting, craft-work, board games, quizzes, topical discussions, toy-making, cooking, jigsaw puzzles, and planning and participating in outings and pub lunches. Often the therapeutic value of these activities is misunderstood. While the focus is on active or passive participation in a particular activity, observation of how patients interact with others is often an indication of their mood. However, the overall aim is to promote well-being and raise morale.

Access to *physiotherapy* in day care may have to be shared by other departments, but for many patients attending day care there is a need for a physiotherapist's assessment, advice and treatment. Their work includes the following:

- teaching breathing exercises and managing panic attacks related to breathlessness;
- giving advice about and treatment and monitoring mobility problems;
- group exercises (often with much laughter, and therefore another morale booster).

Time constraints will inevitably determine the level of input that is possible from a physiotherapist whose workload is shared by other departments. Many day units, recognising this (especially those which are independently funded), employ their own physiotherapist.

The role of the *occupational therapist* in day care will often dovetail with that of the physiotherapist in their common goal of helping patients to cope with activities of daily living. They are able to identify those patients who are at risk from accident or injury, and to provide appropriate advice and equipment to minimise those risks. The practical aspects of their work are underpinned by promoting independence and self-confidence. The cccupational therapist will also advise the activities organiser obout appropriate activities for those patients whose physical abilities are compromised.

Most day units have access to a *social worker* to assist with psychosocial, financial and legal matters, particularly relating to families, children and bereavement care.

All day units have the services of a *chaplain*, and anyone in need of spiritual care has the opportunity to speak to them if they wish to share their concerns, regardless of their culture or beliefs. The chaplain usually liaises (if desired) with leaders of other denominations and faiths, in order to meet individual spiritual needs.

Other therapies that are gaining importance include sculpture, art therapy, creative writing, music therapy, reminiscence therapy and pet therapy. Occasionally the patient's day will include visiting musicians, choirs, artists, and people demonstrating various crafts.

Continuing care

When a patient is discharged from hospice in-patient care, it is helpful for programmes of care and clinical surveillance to continue in day care. In many instances, clinical or social crises are averted and inappropriate admission to hospital avoided. Continued care via hospice day-care services may well alleviate patient and family anxiety.

An increasing number of independently funded hospice day units, after negotiation with the Pathology Department at their local hospital, are offering to collect pathological specimens for analysis. The advantages of this are that treatment can be initiated or monitored quickly, with minimum inconvenience to the patient.

Day units which have medical support from an in-patient service are increasingly able to include medical procedures as part of their services (e.g. 'top-up' blood transfusions, 'tapping' of pleural effusions and ascites, or giving intravenous injections or infusions). These procedures are more likely to be available in a day unit which is funded wholly or partly by the National Health Service.

Many day units are expanding their service to include out-patient services, 'drop-in' facilities for support and information, young people's days and self-help groups, all facilitated by the day-unit team, generally on an appointment basis. *Lymphoedema* treatment can be managed under this system.

Conclusion

Hospice day care is an *enabling* service. It aims to promote health, well-being, support, independence, diversion, creativity and self-esteem, as well as allowing people to remain at home during their care.

Chapter 11, Section 3:   Questions

1 Who compiles the *Directory of Hospice Services in the UK and Republic of Ireland?*
2 Who can refer a patient to hospice day care?
3 Give two examples of referral criteria.
4 Give three examples of complementary therapies and state why they are used?
5 What is the role of the hospice social worker?

References

1   McDaid P (1995) Day care. In: J Penson and R Fisher (eds) *Palliative Care for People with Cancer* (2e). Edward Arnold, London.

2   Russell P (1996) Medical staffing in the day centre. In: R Fisher and P McDaid (eds) *Palliative Day Care*. Edward Arnold, London.

3   Copp G, Richardson A and McDaid P (1998) A telephone survey of the provision of palliative day care services. *Palliative Med.* **12**: 161–70.

To learn more

Fisher R and McDaid P (eds) (1996) *Palliative Day Care*. Edward Arnold, London.

McDaid P (1995) Day care. In: J. Penson and R Fisher (eds) *Palliative Care for People with Cancer* (2e). Edward Arnold, London.

Chapter 11, Section 3:   Answers

1 The Hospice Information Service at St Christopher's Hospice, London.
2 Any healthcare professional who is involved with the patient's care can refer a patient.
3
  - Patients who are *physically* isolated or incapacitated due to their illness or treatment.
  - Patients who are *emotionally* isolated or incapacitated due to their illness or treatment.
  - Patients who are having difficulty adjusting to the changes in their role, status or function within their family or in society.
  - Family stress due to the patient's illness and changes in their role, status or function.
  - Anticipation that future help may be needed by members of the PHCT to manage the patient's care at home, or to cope with family issues or abnormal bereavement.
4 Aromatherapy, acupuncture, reflexology, reiki healing and shiatsu. They are used for relaxation, and for relief of aches and pains and stiff joints, and all aim to promote a feeling of well-being.
5 To provide psychosocial care, and to give advice on financial and legal matters, particularly in relation to families, children and bereavement care.

CHAPTER 12

Integrated care pathways

John E Ellershaw

Introduction

When a patient presents with a problem (e.g. pain), the healthcare professional involved responds by assessing the symptom and suggesting the most appropriate intervention (e.g. analgesics). This in itself appears to be a routine process, but what of the outcome of the intervention? How do we measure whether the treatment prescribed has actually helped? and what do we do if it has not?

Box 12.1: Self-assessment questions

Assess how successful your interventions for symptom control (e.g. pain), have been for:

- individual patients;
- all patients over the past year.

This set of questions begins to challenge how we measure the outcomes of care. Increasingly, we are being asked to demonstrate clinical effectiveness.[1,2] This is not only about the process of delivery of care, but also – importantly – about the outcomes of care.

Within palliative care, the philosophy of care is patient centred and acknowledges the importance of dealing not only with the physical aspects but also with the psychosocial and spiritual dimensions of care.

If then we are to measure outcomes of care, is this not too complex a task to undertake? A number of tools have been developed that examine some or all of the domains of care, and others attempt to measure the patient's 'quality of life'.[3] Many of these tools are additional to the already considerable workload of healthcare professionals, and few of them have been incorporated successfully into everyday practice. Does this therefore suggest that palliative care is special and we are trying to measure unmeasurable outcomes?

This is one conclusion that we may draw. However, there are problems associated with it. First, it invites criticism that if we cannot demonstrate the outcomes of our care, then we are unable to highlight areas of effective practice and other areas that could improve patient care with further education, resources and/or research. Secondly, if funding of services is directed to areas of clinical effectiveness, as demonstrated by outcome measures, then palliative care might find itself well down the priority list.

Therefore there are good reasons to suggest that measuring outcomes in palliative care is worthwhile. What role then, if any, do integrated care pathways (ICPs) have in meeting this need.

What is an ICP?

ICPs have been developed and established in the North American healthcare system, and more recently have been adopted in the UK.[4,5] They are used in a wide range of conditions outside palliative care, including chest pain, breast disease and leg ulcers.[6,7] ICPs provide guidelines and appropriate supporting documentation is included in the pathway for reference. The ICP is central to the patient's care, and is completed by all healthcare professionals involved with the patient. Thus it replaces all other documentation.

How are ICPs initiated?

To undertake the development of an ICP for a whole service (e.g. palliative care) is an ambitious goal. It is advisable to start by identifying an episode or part of patient care that can be developed into an ICP. Following the implementation of an ICP for part of a service, it then becomes easier to develop additional ICPs that link together. For example, in palliative care an ICP for the dying patient has been developed[8] to encompass the last days/hours of life. Following successful implementation of the ICP of the dying patient, it is then possible to develop an ICP for initial assessment of palliative care patients and their ongoing review.

Once a discreet part of a service has been identified for ICP development, all professionals involved in care of the patient during that episode must meet to identify the goals of care. It is essential that all disciplines are involved at this stage of development and have ownership, otherwise implementation will be far more difficult. When developing an ICP for the dying patient, this would include nurses and doctors as the core team, but it might also include chaplains, social workers, occupational therapists and physiotherapists, depending on local circumstances.

How to write an ICP

It is important that an ICP is locally owned. Although there is value in reviewing other care pathways that have been developed, adaptation and further development will be necessary to render them appropriate for local use. The first step is to identify achievable goals, referred to as 'outcomes of care'. This is done by retrospective review of case-notes and by discussion within the team to identify the key outcomes of care.

In care of the dying these 'outcomes of care' can be categorised into the following three phases of care:

1 initially when the patient is identified as being in the dying phase (e.g. the healthcare workers have agreed that the patient is dying and has only hours or days to live);
2 ongoing care of the dying patient;
3 care of relatives after death.

Box 12.2:   Self-assessment question

Consider the last three palliative care patients for whom you have provided care, and identify the key outcomes of care for the first phase (e.g. when the patient is identified as dying).

An example of outcomes of care for this phase is given in Box 12.3.

Box 12.3:   Initial asessment – outcomes of care

Comfort measures:
Goal 1: Current medication assessed and non-essentials discontinued
Goal 2: PRN subcutaneous medication written up as per protocol
            (pain, agitation, respiratory tract secretions)
Goal 3: Discontinue inappropriate interventions
            (blood tests, antibiotics)

Psychological insight:
Goal 4: Insight into condition identified for patient
Goal 5: Insight into condition identified for carer
            (carer understands that the patient is dying)
Religious support:
Goal 6: Religious needs identified/discussed with patient/carer

Communication:
Goal 7: Plan of care explained and discussed with patient/family/other
Goal 8: Family/others express understanding of plan of care

Adapted from the Liverpool Care Pathway for the Dying Patient.

When identifying key outcomes of care, national/local guidelines and research-based evidence should be utilised and incorporated whenever possible. Having identified the key outcomes of care, 'prompts' that enable the outcome to be 'achieved' or 'not achieved' (e.g. a variance) are added beneath each goal. Box 12.4 gives an example of an outcome (Goal 2) and supporting prompts in the initial assessment section of the ICP.

Box 12.4:   Example of Goal 2 from initial assessment section in the ICP for the dying patient

Goal: PRN subcutaneous medication written up for list below   Yes ☐   No ☐
(see attached guidelines for guidance)

Pain:	analgesia	Yes ☐	No ☐
Agitation:	sedative	Yes ☐	No ☐
Respiratory tract secretions:	anticholinergic	Yes ☐	No ☐

Adapted from the Liverpool Care Pathway for the Dying Patient.

This initial writing of the ICP takes at least three meetings. It is advisable to have a facilitator with some knowledge of pathway development in order to complete the development phase as effectively as possible. To increase ownership of the final document, it is important to circulate the draft document as widely as possible among the healthcare professionals who are ultimately going to use it for comment. It is helpful to amend the ICP following consultation, but there is no such thing as a perfect or definitive ICP. An important feature of using the ICP is that it is constantly undergoing scrutiny and changing to adapt to local need and wider developments.

Implementing an ICP

Figure 12.1 shows the developmental steps from a case-orientated culture to a culture of excellence in clinical practice. Too often organisations leap from step 1 straight to using complex outcome measures (step 5). This is perhaps one of the reasons why so few outcome measures have been incorporated into palliative care practice. By adopting a culture that moves towards outcome-based practice (e.g. by the development of ICPs), more complex outcome measures can then be incorporated into the ICP. For example, we may decide to have as a goal for initial assessment in palliative care the fact that the patient is 'pain free'.

Initially we can record a basic measurement (e.g. whether pain is present or absent). However, it may then be possible to incorporate more complex measurements (e.g. a visual analogue scale, VAS) into our assessment. Future analysis will then give a more accurate reflection of the patient's pain control and how it changes over time.

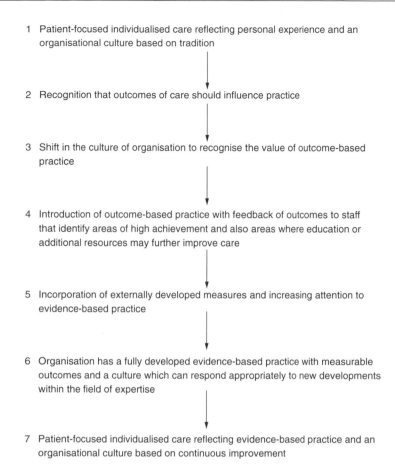

1 Patient-focused individualised care reflecting personal experience and an organisational culture based on tradition

2 Recognition that outcomes of care should influence practice

3 Shift in the culture of organisation to recognise the value of outcome-based practice

4 Introduction of outcome-based practice with feedback of outcomes to staff that identify areas of high achievement and also areas where education or additional resources may further improve care

5 Incorporation of externally developed measures and increasing attention to evidence-based practice

6 Organisation has a fully developed evidence-based practice with measurable outcomes and a culture which can respond appropriately to new developments within the field of expertise

7 Patient-focused individualised care reflecting evidence-based practice and an organisational culture based on continuous improvement

Figure 12.1   Development steps towards outcome-based practice.

The time taken to change the culture of an organisation may range from months to years, and must not be underestimated if the implementation of the ICP is to be effective.

Associated guidelines

In the writing of the ICP, national/local guidelines and research-based evidence should be incorporated whenever possible. It may also be considered helpful by the team to attach key guidelines to each pathway for reference. For example, in the care of the dying pathway, reference guidelines[9-11] would include the following:

1 converting oral morphine to the subcutaneous route;
2 prescribing of anti-cholinergic drugs for respiratory tract secretions;
3 prescribing of medication for terminal agitation.

These guidelines that are agreed upon by the team (which may include a community trust, perhaps with input from the local hospice/palliative care services) are then available to all healthcare professionals involved in the patient's care. This includes new members of staff and locum agencies.

Variation from the pathway

One of the criticisms voiced against the ICPs is that it is a rigid format that does not allow for individualised care. If this were the case, then ICPs would have a limited role in palliative care. In order to address this issue it is important to understand the role of 'variances'. A variance when used in the context of ICPs is a variation from the identified ICP plan of care.

Variances can be either avoidable or unavoidable. For example, in initial assessment of the ICP for the dying patient, goal 5 is to 'ensure that the relative(s) understands that the patient is dying'. If this is not achieved by the healthcare professional, it is recorded as a variance, and the reasons why the outcome was not achieved are also recorded. An unavoidable variance would occur if the patient had no relatives. A potentially avoidable variance could arise if the healthcare professional did not feel confident about discussing death and dying with the relatives.

Information generated from ICPs and the feedback loop

There are a number of ways in which ICPs can be analysed. It is important for an organisation implementing ICPs to identify adequate resources for analysis and feedback to staff. If this is not achieved, staff completing the ICPs will lose enthusiasm, as they will see no benefit to patient care by completing the ICPs.

Analysis includes overall level of achievement of goals followed by either full or selective analysis of variance. For example, in the case of the goal of 'prescribing drugs', an achievement of 95% would indicate a high level of achievement. However, analysis of the variance in the remaining 5% may identify a small change in practice that would lead to further improvement, whereas an achievement of 30% would indicate a low level of achievement, and analysis of variance might reveal that a major change in practice (e.g. access to drugs or a change in prescribing habits) needs to be undertaken.

Feedback to the staff involved in completing the ICP reinforces good practice and enables for discussion and development of alternative strategies in areas of low achievement. In doing so, it is a continuous programme of developing and ensuring clinical excellence.

The opportunity to identify and facilitate educational issues in palliative care

One of the key aims of specialist palliative care teams is to promote the palliative care approach among all healthcare professionals. ICPs can be used as an educational tool both to demonstrate best practice and to link theory with practice. They empower the healthcare professional by giving them access to specialist guidance and knowledge in the form of the ICP document that guides and informs their care.

If generic staff are then enabled to deliver the palliative care approach, this theoretically gives more time to the specialist services to direct their activity towards education rather than direct patient care. Areas of educational need will be identified by analysis of the variances from the ICPs (e.g. communication skills and prescribing), and teaching programmes can be developed accordingly.

Conclusion

ICPs are one potential solution for shifting the culture of an organisation to an outcome-based model. In palliative care they can provide a format for multiprofessional notes and decrease the amount of documentation that is needed by the team. Care pathways can empower generic healthcare workers in the palliative care approach, providing appropriate guidelines and guidance with care at the clinical interface. Analysis of ICPs enables the achieved levels of outcomes of care to be measured, and analysis of variance identifies areas of educational and resource need. ICPs should be seen as an opportunity to achieve clinical excellence in palliative care.

References

1   Glanville J, Haines M and Auston I (1998) Finding information on clinical effectiveness. *BMJ.* **317**: 200–3.

2   Thomson R (1998) Quality to the fore in health policy – at last. *BMJ.* **317**: 95–6.

3   Higginson I (1992) *Quality, Standards, Organisational and Clinical Audit for Hospice and Palliative Care Services.* National Council for Hospice and Specialist Palliative Care Services, London.

4   Overill S (1998) A practical guide to care pathways. *J Integrated Care.* **2**: 93–8.

5   Campbell H, Hotchkiss R, Bradshaw N and Porteous M (1998) Integrated care pathways. *BMJ.* **316**: 133.

6   Zander K and McGill R (1994) Critical and anticipated recovery paths: only the beginning. *Nursing Management.* **25**: 34–40.

7   Kitchiner D, Davidson C and Bundred P (1996) Integrated care pathways: effective tools for continuous evaluation of clinical practice. *J Eval Clin Practice.* **2**: 65–9.

8   Ellershaw J, Foster A, Murphy D *et al.* (1997) Developing an integrated care pathway for the dying patient. *Eur J Palliative Care.* **4**: 203–7.

9   Twycross R (1997) *Symptom Management in Advanced Cancer* (2e). Radcliffe Medical Press, Oxford.

10   Working Party on Clinical Guidelines in Palliative Care 1997) *Changing Gear – Guidelines for Managing the Last Days of Life in Adults.* National Council for Hospice and Specialist Palliative Care Services, London.

11   Adam J (1997) The last 48 hours. *BMJ.* **315**: 1600–603.

PART FOUR

Working together and making it work

CHAPTER 13

Communication

David B Cooper

Pre-reading exercise

Consider the following question before reading this chapter. When you have read the chapter, consider the second question again to see whether you could implement any changes that would improve the problems you identified in question 1.

1 When was the last time you wished communication within or outwith your team could be improved?
2 What steps do you think *you* could have taken to improve the communication problem?

The impact of verbal communication between the health and social care professionals cannot be over-emphasised. Communication is the master key – it fits all locks and opens all doors. How professionals share important and routine information related to the care of the individual, and those significant others within the individual's environment, can and does have a major impact on the successful outcome of any therapeutic intervention.

This chapter will not be laden with references. It merely puts into perspective and provides a rationale for the common courtesy and practice that is part of the professional's daily life. We become so familiar with such communication that it is easy to over-simplify its importance, and consequently we miss the considerable value it holds for individuals and groups alike.

The health professional's life is hectic and full of twists, turns and manoeuvres. Consequently, it is easy to become enclosed within what we have to do – that is, the tasks of daily work. Therefore it is easy to forget to inform other professionals and organisations involved in the patient's care about matters that impinge on that individual's day. If this situation is left unmanaged, then communication breaks down and ill feeling and rivalry can ensue. When one is busy, time is of the essence – and is considered precious and valued. Visiting the patient at home, only to find that the visit has clashed with an unknown out-patient's appointment, can leave the professional feeling frustrated and angry, as if time has been stolen from them.

Consider the following scenario. It is a Friday. Patient M is in considerable pain, and they and their partner have travelled 70 miles on a hot day by car to a specialist clinic. Both of them are anxious about the day, the possible outcome of the treatment, and the patient's future. When seen by the consultant, patient M is advised of a change to treatment for pain control. Patient M, on questioning how to obtain this treatment, is advised that the community nurse will make arrangements with the general practitioner. On leaving the hospital, the patient's partner telephones the community nurse base and a message is left. By now it is Friday afternoon. At 4 p.m., the community nurse arrives at the base, picks up the message and telephones the consultant to find out what medication change he has recommended. However, he has already left. The next telephone call is to the mobile phone of patient M (who is now travelling home) to see what medication has been prescribed. However, the consultant has not told the patient. He had merely said that the community nurse would deal with this matter. The next call was to the general practitioner. The general practitioner and community nurse discuss the best method of pain control available for patient M's need, based on the limited information available to them. It is agreed that patient M should not be left in pain over the weekend, and that the prescription should be left for collection by the community nurse from the surgery at 5.15 p.m. The community nurse contacts the patient again to advise them of the arrangement made with the general practitioner. Patient M and their partner are expecting to arrive home at 6.30 p.m. The community nurse collects the prescription, travels to the pharmacy to collect the drug, and then continues her journey to patients M's home to await their return. The community nurse eventually leaves for home at 8 p.m., 3 hours after the shift should have ended.

To summarise briefly, this case has taken time. Throughout the day the patient and their partner have been left uncertain and anxious about a weekend of pain. The consultant, pressured with work, has progressed through the day unaware of the knock-on effect of the communication, and the problems that this has caused for the patient, their relative and two of his colleagues.

So what happened? At this point one can only speculate. Was the consultant aware of how far the patient had to travel? Was an assumption made that the community nurse was attached to the specialist hospital? What use could have been made of the on-site pharmacy? The obvious solution to this problem would be as follows.

- The patient is given a prescription, together with advice on the use of the drug, from the consultant or nurse attached to the clinic.
- The patient obtains the prescription from the hospital pharmacy.
- A standard form letter (multiple copy) detailing the change of treatment is given to the patient to hand to their general practitioner and community nurse on returning home.

- Normal written communication follows, containing specific details.

Would this be time-consuming? No, as all those individuals involved in the care of this patient are funded by the National Health Service (NHS), the wasted time actually spent would have been reduced, hence cost would be reduced, ill feeling between professionals would be reduced and, more importantly, the patient and their partner would have received effective therapeutic intervention at the correct time and place, and would not feel obliged to apologise to the community nurse for being a source of perceived 'trouble'.

There would be no need for this chapter were it not for the numerous examples of poor and ineffective communication between health and social care professionals, all of which lead to a knock-on effect by reducing the effectiveness of patient care. Other examples include the following:

- the reserved in-patient beds that remain unoccupied because the ward has not been informed of the patient's admission for other health reasons to another ward;
- the community nurse who visits Mr Y, only to encounter a distressed Mrs Y who advises her that Mr Y 'died 2 days ago';
- the wasted general practitioner appointment or home visit, caused by the fact that no one has informed the surgery that the patient has been admitted to a hospital ward. Before there are cries of 'but the family should do that', it should be pointed out that any hospital admission (planned or unplanned) causes disruption and anxiety within a family. Even the most routine of admissions can cause fear, confusion and apprehension. At such times the main concern of the family is for the patient, not the NHS! A simple enquiry as to whether the patient is due to see any other health or social care professional will elicit the information on which the relative can be advised to act, or on which the ward can act;
- the patient who is discharged home without notification of other health and social care professionals involved and, conversely, the community nurse who arranges admission for the patient but who omits to inform her community colleagues or to cancel other hospital appointments.

The above examples occur regularly. As has been made clear, no one profession is to blame. Human nature dictates that we all look for short cuts in order to reduce the perceived workload without consideration of the 'knock-on' effect on others. The consequences of poor communication arise from and affect all health and social care professionals.

Of course, one can communicate with a colleague and still encounter misunderstanding. Anyone with a teenage son or daughter will know that even when the benefits of having a clean, tidy room have been explained for the hundredth time, and a check has been made to ensure understanding of the guidance, numerous reminders administered and the consequences of lack of action explained, the room remains uncleaned. We can only try to improve communication and make our communications as clear and unambiguous as possible. Human nature dictates that some communications will go unheeded or misinterpreted. However, we are not challenging teenagers – we are adult individuals who would all like a good working environment.

During times of pressure and stress, effective communication is the first thing to suffer, yet effective communication reduces both pressure and stress, and effective communication frees up time to deal with other matters that are important to patient care.

Effective communication comes from the top. If senior managers lead by example, then the employee finds the tasks that he or she is set easier to work with and control. However, a lack of such leadership is not an excuse for our own actions, inactions or omissions. Therefore, what form can effective communication take? What can the individual health and social care professional do to improve personal communication with their colleagues?

The following is designed to aid the improvement of communication. In essence, common sense, courtesy and good manners form the basis of good communication. Consider the following as a stepping-stone. Allow for a great deal of personal effort, patience and practice and disappointment, but do keep trying the three 'R's' – Repartition, Repartition, Repartition – as this is the key to success. It is possible to improve communication both as an individual and as a team.

Communicating with a colleague

It is frustrating to feel that your professional communications – the important issues you wish to raise – within and outwith the team at senior, peer or subordinate levels are not being heard and acted upon. It is essential to remember that communication is a two-way process. Often information needs reinforcement and clarification. Both parties need to understand what is required, what is said and, just as important, what is not said in order to keep the interaction and the knock-on effect on patient intervention running smoothly. Do write, do telephone, and do remember to thank people for their actions on your behalf. This is basic good manners, but is often forgotten.

Communicating information

All health and social care professionals receive copious amounts of written communication. It is easy to leave information in the 'in tray' until 'we have more time to deal with it'. Your own personal experience will tell you that such a time never arrives. It is essential to set regular time aside each day to deal with incoming and outgoing mail. If a communication is going to take time to deal with, telephone, e-mail or fax the originator of the communication to let them know when a reply to the communication can be expected. Do not forget to add the date in your diary so that it can be checked and actioned later.

Some individuals within teams withhold information. To possess information that is not yet available to others is often misinterpreted as '*power*'. Practice and service provision can only be effectively improved if information is shared. There is more '*power*' and '*respect*' to be gained from sharing information and resources with colleagues than from withholding it. After all, if no one knows you are holding that information (perhaps on a new treatment method or approach), how can your influence and knowledge over your colleagues be acknowledged? More importantly, how can your colleagues improve patient care?

One way to share information and ensure that it has been read is to circulate the document with a '*circulation list*'. Each recipient signs the list to acknowledge receipt and to confirm that it has been read. To be more effective, individual copies could be distributed.

Regular staff meetings are also essential to smooth the sharing of information. If you are a 'hoarder' by nature, this will be your opportunity to demonstrate your skill and knowledge and at the same time bring the rest of the team up to date.

Communicating change

Change in any organisation is unsettling. Half-truth and rumours need little encouragement for dissemination and cause dissatisfaction. It is easier to have all your colleagues on board the ship than it is to stop the ship, circle, and collect those who have fallen overboard, even if the ship is the Titanic! Change affects all members of the team. To share and be fully conversant with the change, and the process involved, can and does lead to team support. Involvement and a sense of being part of the change process, rather than excluded and unworthy of consideration, is essential for effective communication and ownership of the change (*see* Chapters 14 and 15).

The admission process

Whatever the area of health and social care in which you work, the admission or acceptance of a planned therapeutic interaction with a patient and/or relative will be part of your role. To be effective it is essential that we communicate with any significant others involved in the care of that individual, and the primary worker needs to become the communication co-ordinator. However, this is not to dismiss the importance of all professionals involved in ensuring that communications relating to that individual are effectively dealt with. In the case of emergency hospital admission, often the general practitioner, community nurse, social worker, occupational therapist, community psychiatric nurse or whoever is actively involved in the care is unaware that the admission has taken place.

Even planned admissions can cause communication problems. Other hospital or community care appointments can be missed or the patient may have forgotten to cancel an appointment (e.g. with the general practitioner).

As soon as the individual is engaged with the health and social care professional, information should be collected about other services involved in their care (either directly or indirectly). Planned appointments that may be missed or proposed community visits and/or out-patient appointments need to be noted, and each professional colleague or agency should be informed.

With the patient's permission, information on their past and present health or social problems can be discussed with each agency and a primary worker appointed. Just as important is the information available from the relative(s) (with the patient's permission), relating to the health or social care problem(s) of the patient. Often the patient may forget or feel unable to express important facts and information relevant to the presenting problem.

It is often easier to share information of your involvement with a client using a multi-copy letter. It is good practice (and will be much appreciated by other colleagues) to give the patient a copy of this letter.

The discharge process

If the care needs of the patient have changed since your therapeutic intervention, it may be appropriate to arrange a joint case conference to share valuable information relating to the present and future health and social care needs of the patient.

Withdrawal of professional involvement or discharge should never happen unless adequate arrangements for any continuing care have been agreed and are in place. It is not good practice to withdraw a service or to discharge the patient on a Friday or over a weekend. Crises can and do occur, and community services are not always easily available at weekends. Patients and relative(s) feel vulnerable when intensive services are withdrawn. Even though the patient may require no immediate intervention, there is a sense of safety if it is understood that someone will be available to answer any questions the patient or relative(s) may have should a problem arise. Ten minutes of pre-withdrawal or discharge preparation may save you or another colleague one or more hours of crisis follow-up contact.

It is far more beneficial if the patient knows the name of the community professional or out-patient professional who will be following on care. This is far more reassuring than being told that 'the nurse will call sometime next week'.

The procedure for withdrawal or discharge is similar to admission or engagement. When a date is agreed, a multi-copy letter in a simple 'delete or tick' format can be used to record relevant disengagement or discharge information. This should be posted, faxed or e-mailed to the appropriate professional or agency. Do not forget to give the patient a copy, as this will also help to reinforce the information given verbally about others involved in the ongoing care of the patient.

Avoiding unnecessary cost and time-wasting

For those who will argue that this is additional bureaucracy gone mad, the above guidance, if appropriately acted upon and carefully followed, is cheaper than the cost of a missed appointment or confusion arising from poor communication. A wasted home visit by a health or social care colleague, and loss of money to the patient from a missed appointment with a benefits agency, far outweigh the cost involved in good, effective communication between very busy professionals and agencies. It is likely that you have already been on the receiving end of such effective action. However, you will probably not have recognised how much time you were saved. Indeed, you may not even be able to recall the event(s). However, it is guaranteed that at some stage during your career to date you will on many occasions have experienced the frustration caused by ineffective communication practices. Individual good and bad practices do make a difference, and they do affect others.

Once all health and social care professionals involved in the care of the patient are fully aware of the activities and proposals surrounding the therapeutic interventions on behalf of and/or for the individual, there is a reduction in wasted visits and appointments, telephone contact, repartition of tasks, and time spent chasing up information.

Being aware of other's feelings

Anyone who has made a home visit, only to be greeted by an emotionally distressed relative or friend who informs you that the patient died in hospital, will recognise the emotional distress this can cause the relative(s), friend or carer(s). It has an equal effect on you, the professional. Your greeting may have been inappropriate, you will be unprepared to respond to the relative appropriately, and if the death is not anticipated, or alternatively your professional interventions have been ongoing for a long time and the patient and carer bond is at a deeper level, you may find the news both distressing and upsetting.

There is very little excuse for such ineffective communication. It is insensitive to the needs of the relative(s) and significant others involved in the patient's care, and it can be, and is, avoidable.

If the patient dies in hospital or at home, and you are the community professional involved, it is of vital importance to visit the relative(s) as soon as is practicable. The visit is essential to provide appropriate support and advice, and to commence closure of the relationship in a therapeutic, caring way.

Effective telecommunication

Effective telecommunication simply means making appropriate use of the telephone to communicate effectively with others. The epidemic of the 'I'll call you back' syndrome grows larger every day. Once the immortal lines have been drawled by the overbur-dened professional, you can almost guarantee that you will need to re-establish contact later. In other words, chase the person you called. These four words ('I'll call you back') can have a major impact on patient care, and any effective therapeutic intervention, for either the patient or the health or social care professional on the receiving end of this line of telephone 'cut-off'. It can and does leave the caller feeling undervalued as, invariably, the call is not returned.

We all know how frustrating this can be. If, for whatever reason, you are unable to answer a telephone call or cannot deal with the communication immediately (e.g. because more research is needed before an appropriate reply can be relayed), do remember to phone the caller back. If the query is likely to take a long time, do make occasional progress calls. This acts as a self-reminder to chase up the query, and also lets the originator of the enquiry know that it has not been forgotten or undervalued.

It is useful to bear in mind that it may have taken the individual concerned a considerable amount of effort and courage to make the telephone call in the first place. Whilst the outcome of the conversation may appear routine to you, it could be of vital importance to the patient, their relative(s) or significant others making the call. Equally, it could be you making such a call in future. Would you like to be treated effectively, or would you like to have your query go unanswered and/or be misunderstood?

Setting the example to others

Direction on effective communication comes from the top. If the directive from the senior managers of health and social care professionals is that clear and effective communication is important, then it is likely that the practice will disseminate effectively to the work-force. However, one cannot place all of the responsibility on the boss! Each of us is capable of demonstrating how communication can be effective if we remain cognisant of the part we all play in ensuring that we are understood and heard. We must also exercise carefully the ability to listen to others and analyse each individual's need. Having done this, no therapeutic intervention can take place unless we act on the information we have, and communicate it to others.

A few minutes spent on effective communication now will save time in the future. Misunderstanding, anger, frustration, complaints and worry – not only for the patients and relative(s) with whom we practice, or the other health and social care professionals with whom we come into contact regularly or occasionally – but also for ourselves – can be avoided provided that we communicate effectively.

Why keep walking into doors? Life is difficult enough! We all have a responsibility to make it easier not just for ourselves, but also for others whose lives we touch in one way or another. Effective communication is the master key – it fits all locks and opens the way to therapeutic caring and nursing interventions.

Stress issues in palliative care: caring for the community professional

Robin J Davidson

Pre-reading exercise

A few months ago, a colleague confided in you that she was agitated, sleepless and often tearful in the evenings after work. She is a community nurse and said that in recent weeks three patients, to whom she had been very close, had died prematurely. These people were all around the age of her older sister, who had died of cancer some five years previously. She was drinking too heavily and becoming socially withdrawn, and was about to hand in her resignation. How would you deal with the situation? Spend about 15 minutes answering this question. After reading the chapter, repeat the exercise to see whether what you have read will influence your future approach.

Introduction

Healthcare workers in general and nurses in particular are often hesitant to admit to feeling stressed because of a fear of being labelled as weak, unable to cope or incapable of professional practice. It is therefore important that individuals can understand and detect stress in themselves and their colleagues. The sources and effects of stress among professional carers have been investigated extensively over the past decade.

However, there has not been a particular theme to this work, and for a number of reasons it is sometimes difficult to draw definitive conclusions. First, most of the work has not been based on any particular theoretical framework of occupational stress. Most studies have compared a health service sample with a matched control group or normative test data. Second, there have been very few studies which have employed multivariate methodology in order to elucidate how the various causes and effects of stress are interrelated. Furthermore, little use has been made of qualitative research methods. Third, a wide variety of scales have been used to assess components of stress. Some have been profession-specific (e.g. the Nurse Stress Index), while others (e.g. the General Health Questionnaire or the Hospital Anxiety and Depression Scale) measure psychological morbidity. Sometimes personality scales (e.g. the 16PF) have been employed, as have very specific instruments (e.g. the Coping With Death Scale).

Generally, studies conclude that healthcare professionals show greater levels of stress than matched groups of other workers. However, the variety of instruments used in this research has meant that there have been some problems with consistency across studies. There are also some contradictory findings. The aim of this chapter is to outline a theoretical framework of occupational stress to aid our interpretation of the research. This will be followed by a summary of the sources and effects of stress within a palliative-care working environment. The final section will outline some methods that have been used to develop support systems within palliative care.

Stress and burnout

The concept of stress has been employed in a number of ways. Sometimes it has been used to describe the threats and challenges that confront us, while at other times it is defined as the response to such challenges. However, most workers would now say that the response of stress arises when the demands of our environment exceed the personal and social resources at an individual's disposal. The stress response is multi-factorial, including cognitive, affective, behavioural and physiological components.

- *Physiological* activity in the sympathetic nervous system increases heart rate and respiration, and diverts blood to the muscles which may be needed for the 'fight or flight' reaction. Constant stress can produce psychosomatic pain, fatigue or insomnia.
- *Cognitive* sequelae include excessive worry, racing thoughts, low self-confidence or a sense of hopelessness.
- *Behaviours* such as social withdrawal or excessive alcohol, nicotine or drug use can be used to compensate for this.
- *Affective* disturbance may eventually lead to clinically significant anxiety or depression.

It is now widely acknowledged that stress plays an aetiological role in the entire spectrum of physical illnesses, from the common cold to cancer. A major meta-analysis which reviewed the literature relating to coronary heart disease, asthma, ulcers, arthritis and headaches found stress to be a significant risk factor.[1]

A useful theoretical model is the Person/Environment Fit. This model articulates the interaction between the personal risk factors and the work environment in which the individual finds him- or herself. In the model, stress is viewed as a person–situation transaction in which features of the situation and characteristics of the person combine to influence how the individual is affected by particular stressors. This model is outlined in Figure 14.1.

As the concept of stress is all-encompassing, it is also useful to think in terms of *burnout* for a number of reasons.

1 Burnout is limited to sources of stress in the individual's workplace.
2 Burnout among health professionals has been particularly well researched.
3 Burnout is more precisely defined than stress.

The three components of burnout are emotional exhaustion, depersonalisation and reduced personal accomplishment,[2] and the characteristics of each of these are summarised in Box 14.1. Burnout is said to be a chronic condition, which can lead to deterioration in the quality of care that an individual provides for his or her patients. This may be because of lowered morale, absenteeism, poor physical health or an increase in marital or family problems.

Box 14.1:   The components of burnout

- *Emotional exhaustion*
  Wearing out, depletion of emotional resources, loss of energy, debilitation, fatigue.
- *Depersonalisation*
  Negative, callous, excessively detached attitude towards other people, loss of idealism, irritability.
- *Reduced personal accomplishment*
  Reduction in self-confidence, low productivity, poor morale, inability to cope.

Job risk factors

The importance of the interaction between personal and environmental variables is highlighted in the life events literature. It is not the number of life events that predicts a stress response, but rather how we perceive the events which determines their stressfulness. Divorce may be traumatic for one person and blessed relief for another. Individual factors such as degree of control, personal coping strategies and the extent of social support interact with and can attenuate potential sources of work-related stress. None the less, there are a number of factors that enable us to classify work

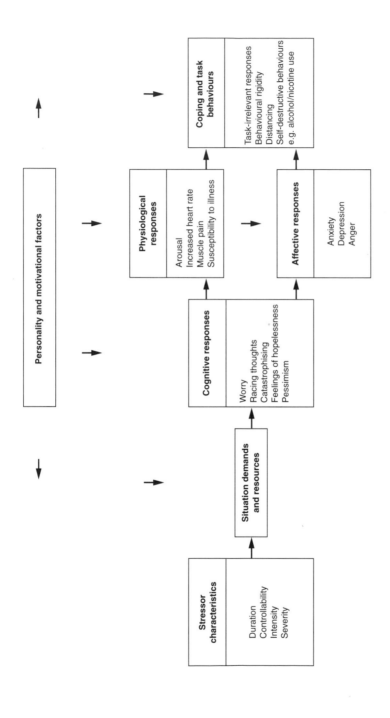

Figure 14.1   Person/environment fit model of stress.

stressors in healthcare environments. These are relationship, task and system maintenance dimensions (Box 14.2).

Box 14.2:   Job-related stress dimensions

- *Relationships*
  Communication problems with managers, lack of team work, conflict with colleagues.
- *Tasks*
  Difficult patient groups, role ambiguity, role conflict, low sense of autonomy.
- *System management*
  Inadequate resources, poor physical environment, old equipment, work overload.

The general literature on stress among health professionals has yielded conflicting findings about the key features of a job which are the major sources of stress. Quantitative questionnaire surveys tend consistently to identify work overload as a major source of stress. However, qualitative research, in which doctors and nurses are asked individually about the most stressful event for them in the previous month, suggests that it is primarily incidents related to death and dying, interpersonal intimacy, and problems with colleagues which are the most prevalent.[3] Complaints of work overload and lack of management support may be used to mask primary sources of stress such as intimacy, death and suffering.

There is little doubt however that a clearly defined role, greater job autonomy, supportive managers, participative leadership, cohesive relationships with colleagues and good working conditions lead to greater job satisfaction, increased performance, higher levels of personal accomplishment and less detachment. In other words, there are a number of consistent features throughout healthcare work environments that can reduce the likelihood of job-related stress or burnout.

There may be some particular job characteristics which can attenuate or enhance stress among palliative care workers. The debate over the past decade centres on the relative importance of these additional task-specific occupational stressors in palliative care. Some would argue that the general sources of stress highlighted above contribute more to job stress than those related to death and dying. Others would disagree, and argue that there are unique occupational stressors in palliative care which override the more typical ones in other healthcare environments.

It has been suggested that palliative care workers are particularly vulnerable to stresses related to over-involvement or sustained intimacy in this highly personalised type of interaction with patients and families.[4] Constantly confronting death leads workers to question how the situation could have been managed better. Home-care nurses have the added pressure of coping without immediate peer support. The so-called *accumulated loss phenomena* have been the subject of some discussion. They are said to arise from continual conflict between the idealised and actual processes of death and dying. Primary palliative care professionals expect to alleviate all suffering, and when this does not happen, it leads to the *ideal* vs. *reality* conflict. Furthermore, those who work with the dying can accumulate apprehension about their own potential losses. It has been suggested that the accumulated grief experienced by palliative care professionals can often result in burnout, particularly emotional exhaustion and depersonalisation.[5] The incremental effect of exposure to the psychological and social pain of terminal illness may gradually reduce the professional carer's sense of self-esteem and self-efficacy.

However, there have been some studies which demonstrate less burnout and anxiety among palliative nurses than among those working in intensive care, oncology and mental health. Furthermore, Vachon concludes her review of the palliative care stress literature by noting that 'while stress exists in palliative care, it is by no means a universal phenomenon'.[6] She goes on to say that stress among palliative care professionals is largely due to the more usual variables such as role conflict, poor communication and isolation from ongoing peer support.

Accordingly, while there may be job-specific stress within palliative care, some of the research literature suggests that this is no greater than that experienced by other healthcare professionals. However, there is a need for more multivariate trials to predict the unique outcome variance of different stressors in the palliative care work environment. There is also some indication that qualitative, single-case studies may accord greater importance to issues related to death and intimacy which are masked in the larger randomised control trials. However, it is clear that there is significant stress within a palliative care work environment, which must be appropriately and effectively managed.

Individual risk factors

There are personal characteristics which can increase the experience of stress among palliative care workers. For example, the literature suggests that there are a number of *demographic variables* which predict stress in this group. It would appear that older, married, experienced workers generally tend to report less stress in a palliative care working environment. However, with regard to experience there are some contradictory findings in as much as a few North American studies found that burnout was correlated with an increased duration of employment in a hospice setting, while this situation is normally reversed in similar UK samples.

There are also a number of *personality variables* which can predispose to work stress. An informative study found that professionals working with dying patients would report less work stress if they scored higher on inner directiveness, existentiality, spontaneity, self-acceptance and capacity for intimate contact.[7] Some *cognitive characteristics* have been shown to protect against stress in palliative care. These include high self-esteem, a sense of personal efficacy and higher levels of assertiveness. From a more psychoanalytical perspective, it has been suggested that people with excessive self-involvement who evaluate self-worth solely on the basis of achievement or material possessions report greater distress in a palliative care setting than individuals whose self-esteem is based on helping others. A number of studies demonstrate that traumatic events outside the work setting, such as unresolved grief, a history of sexual abuse or other ongoing family trauma, have been shown to increase the potential for stress in groups of palliative care nurses. Inadequate preparation and training to enable individuals to deal with the emotional needs of dying patients and their families has also been associated with higher stress levels.[8]

Managing stress

Caring for the carers has only recently received the attention that it merits. The costs in human and economic terms of poorly managed occupational stress are probably incalculable. Workers involved with people who have a terminal illness require sustained commitment, empathic understanding and a high level of intimacy, and if not supported they will show signs of burnout or illness. Individuals do have a tendency to use three types of coping strategies.

1 *Problem-focused* strategies are attempts to confront and deal directly with the demands of the challenge. This involves active problem-solving, planning or other types of more practical activities aimed at overcoming stress.
2 *Emotion-focused* strategies are not aimed at dealing directly with the situation, but rather at managing appraisal of the stress response. Such strategies include acceptance, denial, or trying to reinterpret the situation positively.
3 *Social support* strategies are the most common type of coping strategy, and a number of options for social support are summarised in Box 14.3.[9]

Box 14.3: Staff support options

- Access to a professional mentor for nurses.
- Peer support groups.
- Quality circles that assist in involvement in decision making and teamwork.
- An individual counselling service for those who need more in-depth support.
- Training initiatives to increase awareness.

Support groups can be useful, particularly for primary care professionals who do not have access to informal support in their work. However, support groups are ineffective if they merely become sessions for airing complaints, or if they are not properly facilitated. Basic ground rules for an effective support group include the following:

- confidentiality;
- problems should relate to the work environment;
- the group should not necessarily be used for personal therapy;
- leaders should be experienced in group work.

More generally, there are a number of management interventions that can attenuate individual stress. These clearly include adequate staffing levels, good continued education to improve feelings of self-efficacy, and encouragement to use appropriate anxiety management and exercise strategies. Effective teamwork is essential. It is important that there is a clearly explicit team philosophy, that time is devoted to team-building, and that there are informal and formal mechanisms for team support. Within hospice settings it has been found that teams can grieve more appropriately if procedures such as memorial services, death rounds or memory books are implemented. It is also important to ensure that staff who may have lost a number of patients within a short period of time have access to individual support as necessary.

As well as the more formal support systems, it is perhaps most important that there is a supportive atmosphere among colleagues. In a survey, over two-thirds of a large group of primary palliative care nurses said that talking things over with a colleague was the most useful coping strategy for them. The purpose of any form of staff support is to ensure that carers can maintain their sense of personal effectiveness and self-efficacy. This latter cognitive variable is perhaps most important. When confronted with a stressor, the extent of personal control that we have over the situation plays a major role in buffering its impact. Fisher made the important observation that, within a palliative care setting, it is essential to ensure structured as well as informal staff support in order to facilitate staff grief and provide an environment in which staff can develop.[10] Some people will actively seek support while others may be more reticient about doing so. It is critical that a range of support systems are available which can be tailored to the emotional needs of each individual in the palliative care work environment.

Summary

The consequences of work-related stress in palliative care settings are significant for the professional, the patient and the employer. It is therefore important to identify the sources of stress and to set in place procedures for identification and management of its effects. Burnout is not a synonym for stress, but rather a useful global outcome measure. Although organisational issues are important, there are a number of specific risk factors unique to community palliative care environments that can predict burnout. These can be summarised in terms of the conflict between the idealised and actual processes of death and dying. If support is not available, the accumulated grief can incrementally result in signs of burnout.

Within the palliative care environment, some individuals are at greater risk than others, and it is important that managers are aware of staff members who may be particularly vulnerable. The importance of good communication and ongoing peer support cannot be over-emphasised. Community palliative caregivers represent an increasingly important group of health professionals. It is essential that we understand the pressure they face, and that they are supported appropriately to provide the best possible service to their patients.

Chapter 14:   Questions

1 Which of the following are components of 'burnout'?
   a Emotional exhaustion.
   b Reduced appetite.
   c Loss of libido.
   d Depersonalisation.
   e Paranoid ideation.

2. Which of the following job factors in healthcare settings contribute most to distress as identified in qualitative research?
   a Poor management.
   b Intimacy and death.
   c Work overload.
   d Role ambiguity.
   e Interpersonal problems.

3 Which of the following are affective signs of work stress?
   a Tremulousness.
   b Early depression.
   c Excessive drinking.
   d Chest pain.
   e Worry.

4 Which of the following are accumulated loss phenomena?
   a Personal conflict.
   b Lowered self-esteem.
   c Social withdrawal.
   d Agitation.
   e Aggression.

5 Which of the following are demographic variables which predispose to palliative work stress?
   a Younger age.
   b Lower social class.
   c Low level of education.
   d Being single.
   e Being male.

References

1   Freidman HS and Booth-Kewley S (1987) The 'disease-prone personality': a meta-analytic review of the construct. *Am Psychologist*. **42**: 539–55.

2   Maslach C Jackson SE and Leiter MP (1996) *The Maslach Burnout Inventory* (3e). Consulting Psychologists Press, Palo Alto, CA.

3   Firth-Cozins J (1996) Stress in health professionals. In: A Baum, S Newman, J Weinman *et al.* (eds) *Cambridge Handbook of Psychology, Health and Medicine*. Cambridge University Press, Cambridge.

4   Munley A (1985) Sources of hospice staff stress and how to cope with it. *Nursing Clin North Am.* **20**: 343–55.

5   McKee E (1995) Stress and staff support in hospices: a review of the literature. *Int J Palliative Nursing.* **1**(3): 35–43.

6   Vachon ML (1995) Staff stress in hospice/palliative care: a review. *Palliative Med.* **9**: 91–122.

7   Robbins RA (1995) Death anxiety, death competency and self-actualization in hospice volunteers. *Hospice J.* **7**: 29–35.

8   Power KG and Sharp GR (1988) A comparison of sources of nursing stress and job satisfaction among mental handicap and hospice nursing staff. *J Adv Nursing.* **13**: 726–32.

9   Hingley P and Harris P (1986) Lowering of the tension. *Nursing Times.* **82**: 52–3.

10   Fisher R (1991) Can grief be turned into growth? *Prof Nurse.* **7**: 182.

To learn more

Harris PE (1989) The Nurse Stress Index. *Work and Stress.* **3**: 335–46.

Hipwell AE, Tyler PA and Wilson C (1989) Sources of stress and dissatisfaction among nurses in four hospital environments. *Br J Med Psychol.* **62**: 71–9.

Maguire P (1985) Psychological barriers to the care of the dying. *BMJ.* **291**: 1711–13.

Riordan RJ and Saltzer SK (1992) Burnout prevention among healthcare providers working with the terminally ill: a literature review. *Omega.* **25**: 17–24.

Vachon ML (1995) Staff stress in hospice/palliative care; a review. *Palliative Med.* **9**: 91–122.

Chapter 14:   Answers

1 a and d.
2 b and e.
3 b.
4 a and b.
5 a and d.

CHAPTER 15

Management issues in palliative care: caring for the community professional

Suzanne Mace

Pre-reading exercise

- What can you, or your manager, do to care for the community professional working in your team?
- How can you, or your manager, introduce the changes that you have identified above?

Take 10 minutes to write down your answer, and then read on.

Repeat the exercise after reading the chapter and compare your answers with your earlier responses.

Introduction

This chapter will look at the practical approaches a manager can adopt when offering guidance to a colleague, from either within or outwith the community nursing profession, on staff management and caring for the carer. Throughout this chapter, reference is made to the community nurse and manager. However, it is acknowledged that although the chapter briefly explores the different systems in which the community nurse and manager practise and confront the phenomena of stress and risk in palliative care, *it can and does equally relate to all community profes-*

sionals. Therefore the issues discussed, ideas and suggestions can be applied to *all community disciplines.*

This chapter will:

- identify differences between management and leadership;
- discuss the management of change;
- suggest some effective methods of communication.

It will consider how the manager can respond pro-actively, rather than reactively, in supporting the individual practitioner and/or the team, both within and outwith the immediate care service.

The barriers that slow or block the process of knowledge-led and evidence-based innovation, and ways in which these may be reduced or eliminated, will also be explored. The need for sound education and training will be identified, and consideration will be given as to why the field of palliative care may increase stress. Practical examples of support systems that the manager can introduce when addressing stress reduction will be proposed.

The chapter will also address the following:

- what employees can reasonably expect;
- coping mechanisms that the employer can reasonably expect of employees;
- how support to the manager, both within and outwith the organisation, can be practised effectively.

Community nurse – multifaceted role

The primary role of the community nurse is concerned with the patient. However, integral to this is recognition that there are significant others involved. Such individuals include the family and carers, general practitioners, consultants and other health and social care professionals. The role of the community nurse is an important, integral but small part of the larger picture. As the care of the patient and their family progresses, each professional will take on a larger or smaller role as the skills related to that profession are practised. It is important that this is balanced to meet the needs of the patient with the needs of others involved. A useful framework for helping to conceptualise one's thinking here is the systemic approach. This approach is well documented within the family therapy field (see, for example, Palazzoli and the work of the Milan School[1] and Bowen[2]). Elements of systemic thinking, including subsystems and their interplay, help to clarify the work of the hospice and locate it within the larger picture. If there is a change to one element or member's behaviour, this will impact on, and create a change within the whole system.

For example, given the above, it could be argued that the community nurse working within the hospice is working within three major systems. Figure 15.1 relates to the hospice structure where most community nurses, and the manager, will

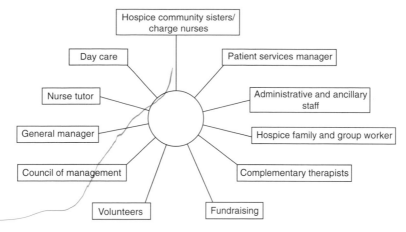

Figure 15.1   Internal hospice system.

meet in palliative care. However, the system shown in Figure 15.1 could easily relate to professional structure within or outwith health and social care:

- the internal (hospice) system (Figure 15.1);
- the external professional system (Figure 15.2);
- the external family system (Figure 15.3).

Although one's professional title and/or role within health and social care may change, the basic principle is the same. However, it is important to remember that each one is interrelated.

Such a diversity of professionals, carers and significant others raises the question of whether or not the community nurse is working in three different cultures that embody different sets of values and beliefs. It also raises the question of the difficulties of having different 'masters', and the dilemmas of where one's allegiance lies.

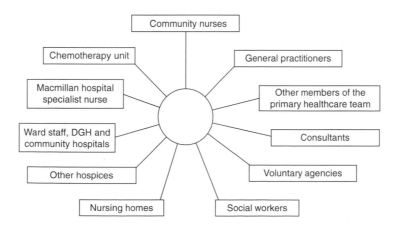

Figure 15.2   External professional system.

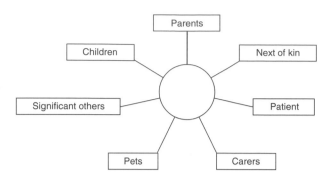

Figure 15.3   External family system.

Confronting the phenomena of stress and risk

When considering the relationship between the patient and the community nurse, there appears to be a tendency not to (or a reluctance to) 'let go' – that is, to discharge a patient when it would be reasonable to do so. The reasons can be varied, and may include the following:

- fear of possible consequences;
- attachment to the patient;
- control of the patient;
- pressures from the patient.

One study which highlighted these issues focused on community nursing and considered the different characteristics of 'long-stay' and 'recently referred' patients.[3]

Part of normal life involves enabling people to take risks, and so it would appear that the problem lies with the worker rather than with the client. If this *is* the case, then one has to ask the question 'is this reluctance to let go an efficient and effective use of our resources?' From a manager's perspective, the answer must be no.

The community nurse is frequently faced with the need to deal with death, and al Quadhi[4] believes that health professionals experience a sense of failure when a patient dies. She suggests that dealing with this is not so much a question of policy, but rather about changing the environment. Therefore staff support is a crucial issue. Although counsellors and support groups have a place, the crucial factor is to develop a much more open culture within the workplace where such issues and feelings may be explored. It is important that staff should feel able to express any sense of failure openly in a non-threatening environment. In this way, it will become evident that they are not alone in feeling such a sense of failure. Alongside this, positive feelings and moments of humour should also be shared. Suggested forums for this to take place include informal meetings with peers, team meetings and clinical supervision, any of which should go hand in hand with continuing education aimed at developing and increasing skills in dealing with stress.

Leadership

A manager may find it useful to conduct a personal audit of the preferred team roles and leadership development in order to identify where, if anywhere, there are short-comings. Such audits highlight areas for action that is necessary to rectify these shortcomings. Two self-examination tools will be briefly mentioned here.

The Belbin Self-Perception Inventory[5]

Scores are applied to eight different team roles:

- implementor;
- shaper;
- team worker;
- completer/finisher;
- co-ordinator;
- plant;
- resource investigator;
- monitor/evaluator.

Belbin[5] suggests that the highest score on team role will indicate how best the respondent can make his or her mark in a management or project team while seeking complementary strengths from within the team when a low score occurs.

The Leadership Development Questionnaire[6]

This examines the inner and outer aspects of leadership in the following four areas:

- managing information and decision making;
- managing resources and planning;
- managing others;
- managing self.

Leadership *vis-à-vis* management

It may be helpful to consider leadership in relation to management. Looking briefly at the differences between notions of management and leadership, Kotter[7] has clearly outlined them as follows: 'It is not true to suggest that leadership is good and management is bad – they are different, but both crucially important for organisational well-being and survival. Management is about producing a degree of predictability and order while leadership is about producing adaptive change'.

Modern theorists refer to management as leadership, but call it transactional leadership.[8] However, recent literature on leadership has drawn attention to leaders who influence their followers' behaviour, and this is referred to as transformational leadership.[9] It could be suggested that leadership in the National Health Service comes from the Chief Executive and Directors, whilst middle managers require good diagnostic skills, sensitivity to subordinates' needs, and flexibility in leadership style in order to react appropriately to changing situations – this is known as transactional leadership.[8] However, the management of health professionals requires a different approach. Konzer and Posner refer to the characteristic inspiring a shared vision.[10] In considering this, it is worth remembering the skills required of leaders. Adair's model of leadership points to the following three areas of need that a leader must look after:

1 task needs;
2 team needs;
3 individual needs.

The key is to maintain a balance between the three sets of needs.[11]

Management of change

The change equation[12] has been referred to in a list of key 'ingredients' for the change process, which is attributed to David Gleicher in Beckhard and Harris's book on change, *Organisational Transitions*, as an equation. The key factors are as follows:

$$f(D,V, S) > R$$

For change to occur successfully, the following combination must occur.

- **D**issatisfaction with the present situation
- **V**ision of a more desirable future and
- the knowledge of the first **S**teps to take in moving towards that future
- must be greater than the **R**esistance to, or cost of, the change.

Health and social services in the UK have undergone considerable changes in the past decade. Such changes, if handled inappropriately, can be destructive, lowering morale and decreasing performance and skills in practice.

In managing change, it is important to select an appropriate strategy and to recognise its strengths and weaknesses. Strategies that may be useful to consider include the following:

- empirical – rational;
- power – coercive;
- normative – re-educative;
- eclectic approach.[13]

Lippitt[14] suggested that the key to dealing with change is to develop a thorough and carefully thought out strategy for intervention, and identified the following seven steps in the change process:

- diagnosis of the problem;
- assessment of the motivation and capacity for change;
- assessment of the change agent's motivation and resources;
- selection of progressive change objectives;
- choosing an appropriate role for the change event;
- maintenance of the change once it has started;
- termination of a helping relationship.

Inevitably there is likely to be resistance to change. Upton and Brooks[12] suggest that the main causes are as follows:

- lack of understanding;
- fundamental disagreement with the philosophy of the change;
- disagreement with different aspects of the change;
- personal loss.

Resistance to change is natural, and it arises for the following reasons:

- preference for stability;
- habit which, once established, often provides comfort and satisfaction;
- conformity;
- threat to economic interest or prestige;
- misunderstanding;
- different perceptions.[15]

Armstrong[15] suggests that people resist change because it is seen as a threat to familiar patterns of behaviour as well as to status and financial rewards. Resistance to change will be less if:

- those affected by change feel that the project is their own;
- the change is seen as reducing rather than increasing present burdens;
- the change has been agreed upon by group decision.

Effective communication

Failures in every area of human society can in general be traced back to a lack of adequate communication. The most important and the least well-used communication skill is that of accurate listening and attending,[16] (to which one could also add checking).

When communicating with the team, a variety of methods can be adopted:

- direct verbal communication;
- indirect verbal communication;
- by writing (letters, individual performance review, reports, memos);
- by the 'grapevine';
- non-verbal communication.

One may suggest that communication between oneself and individuals can often be good, but when those individuals come together, good communications may founder. In such circumstances you may be faced with a blocking of communications.[16] This can take the following forms:

- pairing and colluding;
- distracting and irrelevancy;
- opting out;
- intellectualising;
- 'divide and rule';
- questioning;
- scapegoating;
- the 'put down'.[16]

Education and training

The need for a learning organisation is seen to arise from environmental conditions which create the need for new forms of organisation in terms of flexibility and capacity to respond to change.[17] Certainly, developments in nurse education, including the United Kingdom Central Council's (UKCC) Standards for Education and Practice following Registration,[18] the introduction of the specialist and advanced practitioner roles and the Diploma nurse training, have highlighted this need.

The creation of a learning organisation requires sound education and training. However, barriers do exist which can slow or block the process of knowledge-led innovation. Barriers identified in 1981[19] still apply today.

Nursing is a research-led profession, or at least it should be! The reasons why nurses fail to put research into clinical practice include the following:[20]

- nurses don't know about research;
- nurses don't understand research;
- nurses don't believe research findings;
- nurses don't know how to apply research findings;
- nurses are not allowed to apply research findings.

A useful tool for identifying potential blockages to knowledge-led innovation is the Barriers to Research Utilisation Scale,[21] in which the respondent answers 29 questions concerning barriers to research on a scale of 1 to 4 (where 1 = to no extent and 4 = to a great extent). Having identified the barriers, it is then possible to try to do something to eliminate or minimise them. It is only when specific barriers are identified that we can effectively intervene to reduce or eliminate them or alter clinicians' perceptions of those barriers.[21] The elimination of barriers is an important step towards improving nursing practice through research. and the following are suggested ways of decreasing them:

- maintain a forum for open discussion, meetings and conferences on a regular basis;
- provide essential information at the appropriate time and at level of cognition of participants;
- use a problem-solving approach.[22]

Another approach may be that of addressing the five stages commonly passed through when research findings are successfully adopted. These are as follows:

- knowledge;
- persuasion;
- decision;
- implementation;
- information.[23]

Stress and support

All community nurses face stressful situations. Although some degree of stress is acceptable, occasionally the level of stress exceeds that with which the community nurse can reasonably be expected to cope. It may be that a personal or professional life experience is unresolved or is currently ongoing, or perhaps several professional crises are being experienced at the same time (one stress too many). It may be that a more intense bond has developed between patient and community nurse. This is often unavoidable during prolonged intervention, and everyone is susceptible to becoming more deeply involved as the caring relationship develops. On the other hand, it may be that this is a new experience and coping strategies have yet to be developed. The community nurse's work includes continually forming relationships with dying patients whilst simultaneously preparing for the termination of those relationships.[24]

It is also worth remembering that younger staff have been found to:

- perceive more stress;[25]
- be more prone to burn-out;[26,27]
- report more stressors;[24]
- exhibit manifestations of stress;[24]
- demonstrate fewer coping strategies than older caregivers.[24]

Health and social care professionals can unconsciously project their frustrations on to management, complaining about staff shortages, too many demands being placed on them, and feeling undervalued.[28] However, it is worth remembering that these frustrations may be compounded by the nature of the work in palliative care. Therefore, the manager needs to explore these frustrations carefully in order to identify and effectively manage such situations.

In the face of excessive stress, it is important to identify and implement ways of reducing the latter. Practical examples of support systems that the manager can intro-duce, and which employees can reasonably expect to be available, include the following:

- regular team meetings;
- clinical supervision – provided on a regular basis – allows the individual to question and reflect within a safe, confidential environment;
- peer support;
- one-to-one meetings with the manager, providing an opportunity for staff to talk about painful issues;
- annual development and review, which has benefits not only for the organisation but also for the individual, not least by providing an opportunity to influence individual training and development;
- an effective human resource strategy;
- appropriate policies and procedures which explain the organisation's view of key principles/values and their implications for the work of the organisation.

Equally, employers can have reasonable expectations of employees. One such expecta-tion is that individuals have a responsibility to look after themselves. This includes lifestyle management, such as:

- having outside interests;
- engaging in physical activities and diversions;
- taking time off;
- organising non-job-related social interaction;
- attending to needs for nutrition and adequate sleep;
- meditation and relaxation techniques.

It is essential that the manager establishes and maintains good channels of communi-cation, not only within their own environment but also in the wider system, as sharing and pooling of ideas with other managers are important. Equally, there is a need for clear boundaries to be established. This is essential if scarce resources are to be conserved, whilst at the same time continuing to allow service provision to be effective. Such co-joint practices reduce duplication of effort and avoid any 'treading on toes'. There is always a degree of overlap, but with effective communication this can be reduced.

Conclusion

The complexities of managing a team in any sphere should not be underestimated. Given the additional complexities of managing community nurses working in pallia-tive care, where much of their time is spent in contact with people who are dying, the task may at times seem insurmountable.

Many of the interpersonal skills required of a community nurse are, of course, transferable to the managerial role. However, managers also need to confront other issues, including:

- budgets/finances;
- efficiency/effectiveness;
- contracts/targets.

Managers need to keep a firm hold of the overview, but any move towards fulfilling the service mission and philosophy requires the support of everyone involved in the organisation.

All too often, it is assumed that good practitioners and/or clinicians make good managers. It certainly helps to have the relevant knowledge base and to be familiar with the issues but, to be effective, managers need to take a step back in order to gain a better perspective. Managers also need to work from a clear theoretical base and link this to their practice and the work of the community service. In this way they are able to keep on track and to provide the necessary support in order to reduce the stresses with which the community nurse is inevitably faced.

For the manger to act effectively, he or she needs to be able to identify situations that may be stressful, and to act quickly and effectively to reduce the level of stress being experienced. In some cases, this may mean spending time in individual discussion and listening to the experiences of the community nurse. It may involve professional support – *mutual sharing* – confirming that all that could be done has been done. For others, it may mean guidance on how to deal more effectively with such situations should they arise in the future. It may be necessary to make direct contact with another professional's manager to discuss a more effective response *from both services*. This will often involve compromise on both parts to ensure that effective working relationships are maintained, and that staff are supported. In health and social care, '*them and us*' management and teamwork are redundant. Only when one adopts a '*we approach*' can therapeutic intervention become effective.

Finally, what may be needed may be as simple, but effective, as holding a box of tissues and giving the community nurse permission to cry in a safe, confidential and controlled environment.

References

1   Palazzoli S (1983) The emergence of a comprehensive systems approach. *J Fam Therapy*. **5**: 165–77.

2   Bowen M (1978) *Family Therapy in Clinical Practice*. Jason Aronson, New York.

3   Badger F, Cameron E and Evers H (1989) District nurses' patients – issues of caseload management. *J Adv Nursing*. **14**: 518–27.

4   al Qadhi A (1996) *Managing Death and Bereavement: A Framework for Caring Organisations*. The Polity Press, Bristol.

5   Belbin RM (1981) *Management Teams: Why They Succeed or Fail.* Butterworth-Heinemann, Oxford.

6   Harwood A (1997) What kind of leader are you? *Nursing Times.* **93**: 66–9.

7   Kotter J (1990) *A Force for Change: How Leadership Differs from Management.* Free Press, Oxford.

8   Hersey P and Blanchard KH (1972) *Management of Organisational Behaviour.* Prentice-Hall, Englewood Cliffs, New York.

9   Bass BM, Avioli BJ and Atwater L (1996) *The Transformational and Transactional Leadership of Men and Women. Applied Psychology: An International Overview.* **45**(5): 35.

10   Konzes JM and Posner BX (1987) *The Leadership Challenge: How to Get Extraordinary Things Done in Organisations.* Jossey Bass, San Francisco.

11   Adair J (1988) *Effective Leadership. A Modern Guide to Developing Leadership Skills* (2e). Pan Books, London.

12   Upton T and Brooks B (1995) *Managing Change in the NHS.* Kogan-Page, London.

13   Lancaster J (1982) Change theory: an essential aspect of nursing practice. In: J Lancaster and W Lancaster (eds) *Concept for Advanced Nursing Practice: the Nurse as a Change Agent.* Mosby Co., London.

14   Lippitt GL (1973) *Visualising Change: Model-Building and the Change Process.* University Associates Inc, San Diego, California.

15   Armstrong M (1983) *How to be a Better Manager.* Kogan Page Ltd, London.

16   Scammell B (1990) *Essentials of Nursing Management Communication Skills.* Macmillan Education Ltd, London.

17   West P (1994) The concept of a learning organisation. *J Eur Industr Training.* **18**: 15–21.

18   United Kingdom Central Council for Nursing, Midwifery and Health Visiting (UKCC) (1994) *The Future of Professional Practice – The Council's Standards of Education and Training Following Registration.* UKCC, London.

19   Hunt J (1981) Indicators for nursing practice: the use of research findings. *J Adv Nursing.* **6**: 198–94.

20   McIntosh J (1995) Barriers to research implementation. *Nurse Researcher.* **2**: 83–91.

21   Funk S, Champagne M and Weise R (1991) Barriers: the barriers to research utilisation scale. *Appl Nursing Res.* **4**: 39–45.

22   Olson EM (1979) Strategies and techniques for the nurse change agent. *Nursing Clin North Am.* **14**: 323–6.

23   Rogers E (1983) *Diffusion of Innovations* (3e). The Free Press, New York.

24   Vachon MLS (1987) *Occupational Stress in the Care of the Critically Ill, the Dying and the Bereaved.* Hemisphere Publishing Corporation, Washington, DC.

25   Krikorian DA and Moser DH (1985) Satisfaction and stresses experienced by professional nurses in hospice programs. *Am J Hospice Care*. **2**: 25–33.

26   Masterson-Allen S, Mor V, Laliberte L *et al.* (1985) Staff burnout in a hospice setting. *Hospice J*. **1**: 1–15.

27   Mor V and Laliberte L (1984) Burnout among hospice staff. *Health Social Work*. **9**: 274–83.

28   Speck P (1996) Unconscious communication. *Palliative Med*. **10**: 273–4.

To learn more

Armstrong M (1983) *How to be a Better Manager*. Kogan-Page, London.

Belbin RM (1981) *Management Teams: Why They Succeed or Fail*. Butterworth-Heinemann, Oxford.

Bond M (1986) *Stress and Self-Awareness: A Guide for Nurses*. Butterworth-Heinemann, London.

Scammell B (1990) *Essentials of Nursing Management Communication Skills*. Macmillan Education, London.

Upton T and Brooks B (1995) *Managing Change in the NHS*. Kogan-Page, London.

PART FIVE
Special considerations

CHAPTER 16

The special needs of the neurological patient

David Oliver

Pre-reading exercise

Before reading this chapter, consider the following question.

● How does the palliative care of a patient with a progressive neurological disease differ from that of a patient with cancer?

Test your knowledge again when you have reached the end of the chapter.

Introduction

Many chronic neurological diseases have no curative treatment, and thus the aim from the time of diagnosis will be to provide palliative care. There will be specific symptom control needs for each disease process, but the overall palliative care approach will be similar for all patients, regardless of diagnosis. However, there may be differences in approach compared to the palliative care of a person with advanced cancer, and the aim of this chapter is to look at some of these factors that should be taken into account when caring for a patient with a neurological disease. Motor neurone disease (amyotrophic lateral sclerosis) will be used as an example to demonstrate some of these differences.

Diagnosis

Motor neurone disease, like many neurological diseases, is uncommon. Therefore there may be a period of time during which the patient has symptoms but the diagnosis is unclear. This may be very difficult for both the patient and their family, and the aim of the nurse should be to provide support at this time and to facilitate the investigations and the results so that the period of uncertainty is minimised. Delays may cause different emotions to come to the fore, ranging from anger and frustration to denial that there is even a problem. Time may be needed to allow the patient and their family to talk about their feelings and encouragement of this communication and expression of feelings may pave the way for families to cope with the illness as it progresses.

As the diagnosis becomes clearer and the patient and their family are told the news, increased provision of support and listening is important, but it is equally important to allow the patient their own space. They may need encouragement to ask about the disease and its management, and co-ordination with the neurological services is essential. Many neurological centres have specialist nurses who will be with the patient and their family at this time and who can listen, provide support and answer questions, as there is much evidence that patients are often unable to absorb all that is said, and that they need to have the information repeated on more than one occasion. The specialist nurse may be able to liaise with the services in the community so that the care plan is clear and there is an effective way of obtaining further information for the patient and their family if required.

Case 16.1

Mr T, a 48-year-old ex-soldier, had developed problems with slurring of his speech, and six months later he complained of problems with swallowing. Initial investigations were undertaken at a dental department, and only after a further six months was a referral made to the neurologist. He underwent investigation, including endoscopy, brain scan, electromyography and muscle biopsy, until the diagnosis of motor neurone disease (MND) was made after a further two months, and 15 months after he had first noticed the slurring of his speech.

Even when the diagnosis has been given to the patient and their family, they may have very little knowledge of the disease. MND is a rare disease, affecting only 5000 patients in the UK, so most people have not had contact with someone with the disease, whereas most individuals in the population have known someone with cancer and have some idea about the possible progression of the disease. MND is often a completely unknown disease, and unfortunately the information in some of the generally available books on health is misleading and often frightening (e.g. referring to death from choking, whereas this is extremely rare with good palliative care). It is important to allow the patient to obtain accurate information, and the voluntary associations and societies, such as the Motor Neurone Disease Association, are able to provide information, leaflets and help from local support groups or advisors who can visit patients and their families at home.

The role at the time of diagnosis includes the following:

- listening;
- supporting;
- facilitating investigations and results;
- information from neurology services and voluntary associations;
- encouraging communication.

The progression of the disease

After the initial shock of the diagnosis, the patient and their family may need some time to acknowledge and discuss its effects on their lives. There is often no curative treatment for a neurological disease and, at best, treatment may reduce the speed of deterioration or reduce the effects of the disease on the patient. Although MND has no curative treatment, the drug riluzole (Rilutek, given at a dose of 50 mg twice a day, which blocks the action of the neurotransmitter glutamate within the brain) has been shown to extend life for up to several months. However, it is not a cure and there will be later deterioration.

During the early stages, the patient and their family may be facing many losses – some small and some much larger. With MND there may be loss of movement of the arms or legs or a reduction in speech or swallowing. Moreover, there are other subsequent losses – of mobility and ability to continue in employment, as well as communication difficulties. Some losses may be less visible, such as the loss of role within the family, and loss of status or friendships. There may be many small losses which add up in time to an increasing disability and restriction on the patient's lifestyle.

The aim of the carers at this time should be to support the patient and their family with these losses, and to ensure that a careful assessment is made of the patient's abilities and needs. This assessment will need to be multidisciplinary, involving a physiotherapist, occupational therapist, speech and language therapist, dietitian, social worker and other agencies such as the specialist neurological services, the voluntary associations, social services and specialist palliative care services. Many specialist palliative care services will be able to help in this multidisciplinary assessment of patients, especially with MND, and would prefer to get to know the patient and their family during this early stage of the disease, while verbal communication is retained or not too greatly affected.

Careful assessment of all aspects of the patient's problems is essential, and is summarised below.

Physical aspects

These include the following:

- positioning;
- pain;

- dyspnoea;
- dysphagia;
- muscle stiffness;
- communication difficulties;
- constipation;
- oedema.

Positioning

With increasing muscle weakness it may become more difficult to find a comfortable position, and a careful assessment to ascertain the best position for the patient is necessary to ensure that comfort is maintained.

Pain

Although the sensory nerves are not affected, over 70% of patients complain of pain.[1,2] This may be due to muscle cramps, joint discomfort due to abnormal muscle tone around the joint, or skin pressure pain resulting from immobility.[3] The correct treatment can be given after the assessment, namely muscle relaxants for cramp, non-steroidal anti-inflammatory drugs for joint pain, and analgesics (including opioids) for skin pressure pain.[3,4] Physiotherapy may be helpful for maintaining all available movement and reducing discomfort and contractures.

Dyspnoea

With increasing intercostal and diaphragmatic muscle weakness breathlessness may occur. It is essential that all carers remain relaxed and help to reduce any anxiety, which may exacerbate the dyspnoea. Opioid medication can be very helpful,[4,5] and consideration may be given to ventilatory support. The latter may be non-invasive ventilation using a facemask or, in extreme circumstances and only after very careful assessment and discussion, tracheostomy ventilation.

Dysphagia

This may occur, and an assessment by a speech and language therapist will be very supportive in planning the management of the swallowing difficulties. Careful feeding and alteration of the consistency of foods to aid swallowing can be very helpful. A percutaneous endoscopic gastrostomy (PEG) may be considered, and can be beneficial in reducing the stress of feeding. The advice of a dietitian should be requested.

Mr T developed increasing swallowing difficulties, and both he and his wife were anxious that his diet was inadequate. A PEG was inserted, and within a few days his swallowing and dietary input improved, as the anxiety related to meals was reduced because if he was unable to take food the PEG could be used instead. He continued with an oral diet for a further two years, and then needed to slowly increase the feeding by PEG, as the oral route became more difficult. He was fed almost entirely via the PEG for the last few months of his life.

Communication difficulties

Speech may be affected if the innervation of the head, neck and respiratory muscles becomes affected. Speech may initially sound slurred but may deteriorate greatly, becoming unintelligible due to oral muscle weakness.

It is always important to listen carefully to the patient, allowing them sufficient time to speak, and not interrupting or finishing their sentences. The speech and language therapist will be able to assess and advise on communication difficulties, and aids may become necessary, ranging from simple aids (e.g. a pad and pencil), to small portable aids (e.g. a Lightwriter), or complex computer systems. Other members of the caring team should become familiar with these aids, but again it is important to ask the patient one question at a time, giving them time to communicate and use these alternative communication systems.

Other symptoms

These may include constipation, anxiety, depression, hunger and muscle stiffness, and all of them will require careful multidisciplinary involvement. It is essential for the team to meet on a regular basis so that the care and the equipment offered are co-ordinated. It is also important to ensure that the patient and their family are not overwhelmed by the number of carers, and that they do not become confused by the complexity of the number of professionals visiting them.

Psychosocial aspects

These include the following:

- diagnosis;
- prognosis;
- physical and mental changes;
- fears;
- progression;
- sexuality.

Anyone facing a progressive neurological disease will have fears and concerns, as will their family. Sources of fear and anxiety include the following:

- the disease itself – they may know little themselves and read misleading information in health-related books;

- the progression of the disease and fears about becoming disabled and dependent;
- the prognosis, and fear of the process of dying or death itself;
- other physical or mental changes – there may be fears of mental deterioration. Although this may occur in some neurological conditions (e.g. dementia in multiple sclerosis and Huntington's disease), in MND confusion is rare;
- sexuality – patients and their families may find it difficult to discuss these issues, but studies have shown that if the nurse or other carer is willing to talk about sexuality without embarrassment, patients have many concerns that they want to discuss. In MND, sexual function is usually unaffected, but couples may need advice and permission to cope with the difficulties and changes that occur due to increasing disability. Advice on the use of different positions or the use of mutual masturbation may be very helpful.

    One patient in a survey of sexuality and MND wrote 'thank God *that* isn't a muscle' and described how helpful it had been that a nurse had discussed sexuality with him and his partner as a couple and encouraged them to experiment and continue with the sexual aspect of their relationship.

The family of a patient with a neurological illness needs support, advice and help. They will have their own concerns, which may be very different from those of the patient.

- They may have their own fears of the illness. For instance, the families of patients with MND often fear – unnecessarily – the terminal stages of the disease progression. They may also fear the development of the disease themselves.
- Communication may be difficult. Patients with a neurological illness may experience particular communication problems, as the motor speech mechanisms can be affected by the disease process – ranging from changes in the brain (e.g. as with a cerebral tumour), causing alteration in the patient's language or word-finding abilities (dysphasia), to difficulties caused by weakness of the muscles of the head and neck (e.g. as in bulbar palsy of MND), or a mental deterioration which affects the ability to communicate (e.g. as with dementia). Support of both the patient and their family is essential to help them to cope with these difficulties, and the wider multidisciplinary team approach may be very helpful, involving the speech and language therapist at an early stage in assessing and then maintaining communication skills. Communication aids, such as a spelling board or more sophisticated computer systems, may be of great benefit in helping a patient and their family to continue to communicate. There may be communication difficulties within the family, and they may need support and encouragement to share their feelings together. Facilitation of this by the professional carers can be very helpful.
- Finance – the care of a severely disabled person may necessitate the spouse or partner leaving their employment, and financial problems can easily ensue. Advice from a social worker or care manager may help to reduce these stresses.
- Children – many families may try to exclude children and grandchildren from involvement with the patient and the disease, hoping to protect them from distress. However, children of all ages will realise that all is not well, although the extent of

their knowledge will depend on their age, maturity and previous experiences. It is helpful to encourage families to include the children, and the help and advice of a social worker may be invaluable in helping both the parents and the children to talk about the illness and the future. Informing and involving the school will also be helpful, so that everyone is aware of possible stresses on the children.

• There may also be very difficult decisions for families to consider when someone has a neurological illness. These may include decisions about continuing or ending treatment regimes, such as enteral feeding or ventilation. Support for families is essential, as although the ideal may be for the patient and their family to be involved in the decision-making process, this may not always be possible if the patient is no longer capable of decision making. There may also be conflicts between the views of the their patient and family, or between different members of the family. Close involvement and discussion with families is important, so that they feel not only involved but also included in the decision-making process, without necessarily experiencing the burden of being the only ones to make the decision.

The carers will need to be open to these concerns of the patient and their family, and to listen carefully to what concerns them. Never assume what is affecting them. The wider multidisciplinary team will need to be open to these concerns, and a social worker or family counsellor may be particularly effective in helping a patient and their family to cope with all of these changes and fears.

Spiritual aspects

Patients may have many other concerns of a more spiritual nature, such as asking the questions 'why me?' or 'what is going to happen to me when I die?' Listening is essential, and a dogmatic approach should be avoided. There are no easy answers, and time spent listening to the patient and allowing them to share the concern may be sufficient. More specialised help from a religious leader, psychologist, social worker or counsellor may also be necessary. (Spirituality is discussed further in Chapter 9.)

Disease progression

Assessment as the disease progresses includes:

• listening;
• multidisciplinary co-ordinated care;
• involving the patient and their family;
• symptom assessment and control;
• remembering all aspects of care (physical, psychosocial and spiritual).

Specialist palliative care services may become involved in the care of patients during the early stages of the disease, or as deterioration occurs.

- The advice and support of the multidisciplinary home care team is very helpful in the care of the patient and family.
- Day hospice care allows for family respite, multidisciplinary assessment, socialisation for the patient and specific help (e.g. physiotherapy or occupational therapy).
- In-patient care may allow for the multidisciplinary assessment of symptoms, respite for family, or rehabilitation.
- The hospital palliative care team provides advice and support in hospital.

The involvement of the specialist palliative care multidisciplinary team will help to facilitate the care of the patient. However, other teams may be involved, including the specialist neurology team, disability team and voluntary groups (e.g. as the MND Association). It is essential that there is co-ordination, and the primary healthcare team has a very important role in ensuring that there is continuity of this collaborative care.

Many other disciplines may be involved in the co-ordinated care of the patient and their family, including the following:

- nurses (specialist neurology nurse, specialist palliative care, e.g. Macmillan nurse, community nurse);
- medical staff (consultant neurologist, rehabilitation consultant, palliative medicine consultant);
- physiotherapist;
- occupational therapist – hospital and Social Services;
- social worker/clinical psychologists/counsellor;
- speech and language therapist;
- dietitian;
- chaplain/religious leader;
- representative from specialist voluntary support agency (e.g. MND Association);
- care manager from Social Services.

With so many professionals involved in the care of the patient and their family, it is essential to have regular meetings to co-ordinate care. It has been suggested that a 'key-worker' should be defined, who would then be able to ensure that care is co-ordinated and the patient and their family are not overwhelmed by the care provided, but that they are supported and allowed to maintain their independence and control over such care.[6] However, as the patient and family's needs are continually changing, the primary worker may also need to change.

The terminal stages

As the patient deteriorates there is an even greater need to ensure that their symptoms are controlled as effectively as possible and all the concerns of the patient and family are addressed. It is particularly important that all individuals involved in the care of the patient are aware of the deterioration and are able to communicate their concerns. Often the change in the care is not appreciated by all members of the team, leading to confusion over the aims of care, and this in turn can lead to confusion and loss of faith in the caring team.

During this time the patient may be able to fulfil personal aims and make preparations for the future. This could include any of the following:

- visiting friends or family;
- making a will;
- organising the funeral;
- preparing audio-tapes or letters for children or grandchildren;
- ensuring that all of the family finances are sorted out;
- helping family and friends with the grief they may be feeling;
- planning further care, such as considering possible admission to nursing care or a hospice.

These may be very difficult activities for some patients. They may also need encouragement to start or complete them, and the professional carers may have a very important role in encouraging the patient and their family to make the most of the time that they do have left. It is important to allow the patient to remain as active as possible and to continue to be involved in their care and the decisions that may have to be made.

After the insertion of the PEG tube, Mr T was very keen to visit Australia to see his brother who had emigrated there 25 years previously. His family helped to raise the funds by a sponsored parachute jump and pub raffles, and applications were made to various charities and organisations for money. He was able to take the holiday, with his family, and enjoyed the chance to meet with his brother again. He then took further holidays in the Canaries and a fishing trip to Ireland with his friends.

It is also helpful for the carers to be prepared as deterioration occurs. At this time it is important that the team discusses further plans, particularly the following:

- place of care – will the patient be able to remain at home, or should admission to a hospice or hospital be considered?
- is extra help required, such as increased care from Social Services or nursing care, both in the day and at night?
- should medication be provided so that it is available if necessary?

Many patients with MND fear choking and dypnoea, in the terminal stages of the disease. With good symptom control this should not become a problem for the majority of patients. The MND Association has produced the Breathing Space Kit to help to reassure patients and their families. The kit consists of a leaflet on the care that may be necessary in the terminal stages, including a discussion of the medication that may be required, together with a box to hold the medication. After discussion between the patient, family, doctor and nurse, the medication can be provided as follows:

- diamorphine, 5–10 mg (or according to the oral dose), for analgesia;
- midazolam, 5–10 mg, for sedation;
- hyoscine hydrobromide, 400–600 microgramme, to reduce secretions.

This medication is then available and can be given in the event of a crisis, by any professional who may be visiting the patient, and should help the locum or covering professional to know what has been discussed by the patient and family. If the patient improves subsequently, they may be able to return to oral medication, or a continuous subcutaneous infusion administered by syringe driver may be considered. The presence of the kit may provide reassurance and security for both the patient and their family.

Other medication may be necessary to control symptoms, such as analgesics for pain and dyspnoea, muscle relaxants for spasm, anticholinergics (such as hyoscine) for chestiness and anticonvulsants to prevent fits. It may be possible to give this medication orally until near to death,[4,5] but parenteral medication may become necessary, given by regular subcutaneous or intramuscular injection or continuous subcutaneous infusion by syringe driver.[7]

Bereavement

The care of the family in bereavement starts before the death, as the care of the patient and their family throughout the disease progression will influence the bereavement. Encouragement of the expression of feelings between the family members will help the grieving process, and there is a need to be available for families to answer any questions they may have about the death and to support them at this time. If there has been a long period of caring for the patient during a slowly progressive disease, there may be many mixed feelings – of relief at the end of the strain of caring, mixed with guilt at these feelings.[8] Many families are able to work through these feelings by themselves with the support of other family members and friends. Others may benefit from extra help from their general practitioner, a counsellor, clinical psychologist, social worker or psychiatrist.

**Chapter 16:	Questions**

1 Specialist palliative care services may be involved in the palliative care of a patient with a progressive neurological disease:
   a early in the disease process
   b only if there are severe symptom control issues
   c only in the very terminal stages of the disease
   d if the neurologist insists on their involvement.

2 A percutaneous endoscopic gastrostomy may be suggested:
   a only if there are very severe swallowing problems, in the final stages
   b early in the disease process, before there are appreciable problems with swallowing
   c when swallowing is starting to be difficult and the patient is losing weight
   d when swallowing is difficult and meals are becoming a problem.

3 In a crisis when the patient is distressed with their breathing:
   a a doctor should be called and antibiotics given
   b the patient should be turned on their side and suction given
   c an injection of diamorphine with midazolam and hyoscine should be given
   d the patient's family should be excluded from the room so that they do not become further distressed by the situation.

4 When assessing a patient, the sexual needs of the patient and their partner:
   a should rarely be a problem if they are over 60 years of age
   b rarely present a problem as the disability progresses
   c should be addressed sensitively with all couples, regardless of age
   d should only be considered if the patient is in a stable heterosexual relationship.

5 Pain:
   a never occurs in MND as the sensory nerves are unaffected
   b may be relieved by opioids, especially if there is general discomfort
   c may be related to muscle spasm
   d is usually due to some other cause and not MND.

References

1   Newrick PG and Langton-Hewer R (1985) Pain in motor neuron disease. *J Neurol Neurosurg Psychiatry.* **48**: 838–40.

2   O'Brien T, Kelly M and Saunders C (1992) Motor neurone disease: a hospice perspective. *BMJ.* **304**: 471–3.

3   Oliver D (1994) *Motor Neurone Disease* (2e). Royal College of General Practitioners, London.

4   Oliver D (1998) Opioid medication in the palliative care of motor neurone disease. *Palliative Med.* **12**: 113–15.

5   Oliver D (1996) The quality of care and symptom control – the effects on the terminal phase of ALS/MND. *J Neurol Sci.* **139 (Suppl.)**: 134–6.

6   Newrick PG and Langton-Hewer R (1984) Motor neurone disease: can we do better? A study of 42 patients. *BMJ.* **289**: 539–42.

7   Oliver D J (1985) The use of the syringe driver in terminal care. *Br J Clin Pharmacol.* **20**: 515–16.

8   Oliver D and McMurray N (1993) Bereavement – whose responsibility? *Palliative Med.* **7 (Suppl. 2)**: 73–6.

To learn more

Beresford S (1995) *Motor Neurone Disease*. Chapman and Hall, London.

Oliver D (1994) *Motor Neurone Disease* (2e). Royal College of General Practitioners, London.

Oliver D (1995) *Motor Neurone Disease: A Family Affair*. Sheldon Press, London.

Rose V (1992) Understanding motor neurone disease. *Prof Nurse.* **7**: 784–86.

Skelton J (1996) Caring for patients with motor neurone disease. *Nursing Standard.* **10**: 33–6.

Williams AC (ed) (1994) *Motor Neurone Disease*. Chapman and Hall, London.

Chapter 16:   Answers

1 a
2 d
3 c
4 c
5 b and c

CHAPTER 17

Legal aspects of palliative care

Bridgit Dimond

Introduction

It is essential that those who are providing palliative care for patients have a clear understanding of the legal framework within which they work, so that they can respond appropriately to the questions which patients and colleagues may raise. Clearly, this chapter could form a book in itself, and only the basic principles of the law that applies to this area of healthcare can be given. However, reference will be made to books for further reading. The topics to be covered are shown in Box 17.1.

Box 17.1: Topics covered in this chapter

1 Duty of care and accountability in pain management: civil law, employment and professional liability.
2 The criminal laws relating to murder, manslaughter, suicide and euthanasia. The cases of Dr Bodkin Adams and Dr Nigel Cox.
3 The law relating to consent: the autonomy of the competent patient and the right to refuse care.
4 Letting die: the mentally competent adult.
5 Living wills/advance refusal or directive.
6 Letting die: the mentally incompetent adult; acting in the best interests under Re F principle; Law Commission proposals – and who decides?
7 Not For Resuscitation instructions.
8 Record-keeping.
9 Statements.
10 Statutory framework for the provision of healthcare.

Duty of care and accountability in pain management: civil law, employment and professional liability

Pain management gives rise to the same standards of accountability and professional responsibility as every other aspect of healthcare. However, there have been few legal cases in which the harm which is alleged is simply pain, although there are many in which pain represents part of the suffering that has occurred as a consequence of other harm resulting from negligence. Thus if a second operation becomes necessary as a result of negligence during the first one, then the patient suing for compensation will argue that the damages payable must include an amount for the additional pain that resulted from the second operation.

However, the increase in understanding of pain management and the raising of standards of care in controlling pain may well lead to an increase in litigation based on the fact that an individual has, as a result of negligence on the part of the defendant or the defendant's employees, suffered unacceptable levels of pain.

Let us assume that such a situation arises (the possible facts are shown in Box 17.2). What legal consequences could flow to professional staff?

Box 17.2:   A situation giving rise to legal issues

Gwen Roberts is a diabetic controlled by insulin who suffers from severe rheumatoid arthritis which gives her excruciating pain. She has been diagnosed as having breast cancer. In the terminal stages of her illness, she is referred to the palliative care services. Mavis Jones, the community nurse providing the pain management service, sets the syringe driver at the wrong dosage and Gwen receives an inadequate level of pain control medication. In her desperation, Gwen injects herself with insulin and dies. Her distraught family holds the community trust to blame for Gwen's death, and they wish to bring a legal action against the Trust and its employees. What legal issues arise?

An imaginary situation: civil liability

Mavis Jones clearly has a duty of care towards Gwen. This arises both from the laws of negligence (part of a group of civil laws known as torts) and from the statutory duty placed upon the Secretary of State to provide health services. This statutory duty is delegated to health authorities, which have the responsibility with primary care groups of arranging provision of the services, by Trusts and other providers.

To establish that there has been negligence, Gwen's relatives will have to show that a duty of care was owed, that there has been a breach of this duty of care, and that as a reasonably foreseeable consequence of this breach of duty, harm has occurred.

The standard of care

Mavis clearly owes a duty of care to Gwen, and if she has failed to provide appropriate pain relief, because she has wrongly set up the syringe driver, then she is clearly in breach of her duty of care. The determination of whether there is a breach of the duty of care is based on what has become known as the Bolam test (i.e. what is the reasonable standard of care).

> '[A doctor] is not guilty of negligence if he has acted in accordance with a practice accepted as proper by a responsible body of medical men skilled in that particular art. ... Putting it the other way round, a man is not negligent if he acts in accordance with such a practice, merely because there is a body of opinion who would take a contrary view.'[1]

Expert evidence would be used to define what standard of care Gwen would have been entitled to expect, and whether what Mavis did was below the accepted level of care. There may be different standards of care which would be acceptable to a competent body of professional opinion, and the person bringing the action (the claimant) would fail if the defendant was supported by competent expert opinion. The House of Lords recently emphasised that such expert opinion must flow logically and reasonably from the specific circumstances:

> 'The use of the adjectives "responsible, reasonable and respectable" (in the Bolam case) all showed that the court had to be satisfied that the exponents of the body of opinion relied upon could demonstrate that such opinion had a logical basis.'[2]

Applying the Bolam test to the facts of Gwen Roberts' situation, it would be difficult to imagine that any expert could support the wrong setting of the syringe driver as defensible, so there would appear to be – at least at first sight – a breach of the duty of care owed by Mavis to Gwen.

Causation

The relatives would also have to show that Gwen's death was a consequence of this failure. It may be that Gwen was so depressed that there was a danger that she would commit suicide irrespective of the care which was provided (i.e. she would have died anyway and failures by Mavis were not to blame). In this case, the action for compensation would fail.

However, if the relatives can show that Gwen was coping very well and it was the unremitting pain that caused her to become so depressed that she committed suicide, then an action for the negligence which caused harm may succeed.

Vicarious liability

It is of course unlikely that Mavis would be personally sued. The relatives would normally seek compensation from her employers (i.e. the Trust). This is because employers are held liable for the negligence caused by their employees whilst acting in the course of employment. This doctrine of vicarious liability ensures that innocent victims obtain compensation from employers who are required to be insured for public liability. (NHS trusts do not have to be insured for medical negligence, as the NHS carries its own insurance.)

Professional liability

However, Mavis may also be liable before the professional conduct committee (PCC) of the United Kingdom Central Council for Nursing, Midwifery and Health Visiting (UKCC), her registration body. If she is found guilty of misconduct (i.e. conduct unworthy of a nurse, midwife or health visitor), then various sanctions are available to the PCC, with the ultimate sanction of striking her name off the Register.

Liability as an employee

As an employee of the Trust, Mavis has a duty, which is implied by law into the contract of employment, to act with reasonable skill and care in fulfilling her contractual duties and to obey reasonable instructions. It therefore follows that if she is guilty of negligence in relation to the care of the patient, she may also be in breach of the implied term in her contract of employment, and therefore she could face disciplinary action in relation to the care she has failed to provide for Gwen. Disciplinary action can range from a first oral warning to dismissal. If she is dismissed, Mavis could – provided that she has the necessary continuous length of service – apply to the industrial tribunal for a declaration that she has been unfairly dismissed.

It is possible that all three hearings could arise as a result of professional negligence and, in addition, there may be a prosecution.

The criminal laws relating to murder, manslaughter, suicide and euthanasia. The cases of Dr Bodkin Adams and Dr Nigel Cox

Manslaughter

In the situation shown in Box 17.2, Mavis did not intend that Gwen should die, nor is it likely that her actions, although grossly negligent, led directly to Gwen's death, so there could not be a successful prosecution for murder. (It would be different if Mavis had set the syringe driver so that a large overdose of medication took place.) It has been held that if a professional acts with such gross recklessness and negligence as to amount to a criminal act, then there can be successful criminal prosecution for causing the death of the patient. This was established as a principle by the House of Lords in a case where a patient died on the operating table because one of the gas tubes became disconnected. The anaesthetist was convicted of causing the death of the patient.[3]

Euthanasia

This country does not recognise any law of euthanasia. If any person takes action intending to bring about the death of another, that is a criminal offence – murder or manslaughter. It is murder if the perpetrator intended that outcome or acted with gross recklessness with regard to the possibility that death could occur.

Murder is defined as occurring when:

'a man of sound memory, and of the age of discretion, unlawfully killeth within any country of the realm any reasonable creature in rerum natura *under the king's peace, with malice aforethought, either expressed by the party or implied by law, so as the party wounded, or hurt, etc., die of the wound or hurt, etc.'*[4]

The time limit which once existed, whereby the person must die of the wound or hurt within a year and a day, was removed in 1996, so there is now no time limit within which the person must die for murder to exist. There is a mandatory life sentence for anyone over 18 years who is convicted of murder, and the judge has no discretion over the sentence.

The crime of manslaughter covers both voluntary and involuntary manslaughter. Voluntary manslaughter has occured if the death was intended, but special circumstances reduce it legally from murder to manslaughter. These include death following a suicide pact, provocation and diminished responsibility. Involuntary manslaughter exists when the mental intention (i.e. *mens rea*) to cause death is missing. Thus in cases of gross negligence, death may result but there is no intention to kill. Killing recklessly may or may not be sufficient to be murder. If the accused has acted with such reckless regard to the possibility that death might occur from his actions, judged on an objective basis, then a charge of murder may arise; otherwise, a manslaughter charge would be brought. An intention to escape from lawful arrest that results in a death would also be grounds for a manslaughter charge.

Following a verdict of guilty of manslaughter, the judge has the discretion to sentence the convicted person to anything from absolute discharge to imprisonment for a considerable length of time, as well as any order under Part 3 of the Mental Health Act 1983, if the necessary conditions exist. There have been several cases of 'mercy killing', in which a relative has ended the life of a grossly disabled or terminally ill person, where following a conviction for manslaughter the judge has sentenced the defendant to a conditional discharge or probation,[5] with no prison sentence.

Suicide

Suicide ceased to be a crime after the passing of the Suicide Act 1961. A person who has failed in a suicide attempt is no longer guilty of a crime. However, to assist or aid another person in a suicide attempt remains illegal. Section 2(1) of the Suicide Act 1961 is shown in Box 17.3.

Box 17.3:   Suicide Act 1961 Section 2(1)

A person who aids, abets, counsels or procures the suicide of another, or an attempt by another to commit suicide, shall be liable on conviction on indictment to imprisonment (up to 14 years).

The effect of Section 2(1) of the Suicide Act 1961 is that if any health professional or indeed anyone else is asked by a person to assist in bringing about his or her death, and obliges, this is a criminal act. This is so even if the person making the request is terminally ill. It also applies to those who give advice. Thus there were convictions under the Suicide Act of those who printed a book advising people on how to end their lives.

The case of Dr Nigel Cox[6]

Dr Nigel Cox, a rheumatologist in Winchester, was convicted of causing the death of a patient to whom he had administered potassium chloride. He was given a suspended prison sentence. The patient was in crippling pain and terminally ill, and her relatives were concerned about her condition. Dr Cox was also brought before his employers (the Wessex Regional Health Authority) to face disciplinary proceedings, but retained his post. In addition, he was brought before professional conduct proceedings of the General Medical Council, but he stayed on the Register.

The case of Dr Bodkin Adams

In contrast to the case of Dr Cox, Dr Bodkin Adams was acquitted following a trial where it was alleged that he had caused the death of Mrs Morell, a resident in a nursing home in Eastbourne, by giving her excessive morphine.

The trial judge, Mr Justice Patrick Devlin, directed the jury that:

'There has been a good deal of discussion about the circumstances in which a doctor might be justified in giving drugs which would shorten life in cases of severe pain. It is my duty to tell you that the law knows of no special defence of this character. But that does not mean that a doctor aiding the sick or dying has to calculate in minutes or hours, or perhaps in days or weeks, the effect on a patient's life of the medicines

which he administers. If the first purpose of medicine – the restoration of health – can no longer be achieved, there is still much for the doctor to do, and he is entitled to do all that is proper and necessary to relieve pain and suffering, even if the measures he takes may incidentally shorten life. ... It remains a law that no doctor has the right to cut off life deliberately. ... What counsel for the defence was saying was that the treatment that was given by the doctor was designed to promote comfort, and if it was the right and proper treatment of the case, the fact that incidentally it shortened life does not give any grounds for convicting him of murder.'[7]

This ruling still applies today. However, note should be taken of what is 'right and proper treatment'. It could be that a very high dose of morphine would be justified for a patient who needed that level of the drug to achieve pain relief, whereas giving the same dose to a person who had not become resistant to morphine would be lethal and grossly reckless, and would justify a criminal conviction. 'Right and proper treatment' must also take into account current research on effective pain management.

Annie Lindsell, a sufferer from motor neurone disease, brought a court action for a declaration that her GP could administer palliative drugs which could have the effect of shortening her life. She was told that a responsible body of medical opinion supported her doctor's treatment plan, and she then withdrew her application for the court's intervention.[8] She died a few months later.

The law relating to consent: the autonomy of the competent patient and the right to refuse care

A mentally competent adult (i.e. one over 18 years of age) has the right to refuse to give consent to treatment even though that treatment is a life-saving necessity.[9] The Court of Appeal has declared that, provided the individual is mentally competent, he or she does not have to have a good reason – or even any reason – for the refusal, and health professionals must accept it.[10]

Letting die: the mentally competent adult

If a mentally competent adult refuses care, then the health professionals must accept their refusal. This is the patient's right of autonomy.

Although it is a crime to aid and abet the suicide of another, it is not a crime to accept the refusal of a mentally competent adult to receive further treatment, even though this may mean that death could occur.

The law thus distinguishes between withholding treatment from a mentally competent person who has refused it (or – see below – from a mentally incompetent person, where that is in his best interests) and bringing about death in a positive way. This distinction which is drawn in the law between killing a person and allowing a person to die has been criticised by some philosophers,[11,12] who argue that the outcome is the same. However, the distinction is at the heart of the decision made by the House of Lords to permit the artificial feeding of Tony Bland to cease.

Lord Browne-Wilkinson addressed the dilemma as follows:

> 'How can it be lawful to allow a patient to die slowly, though painlessly, over a period of weeks from lack of food, but unlawful to produce his immediate death by a lethal injection, thereby saving his family from yet another ordeal to add to the tragedy that has already struck them? I find it difficult to find a moral answer to that question. But it is undoubtedly the law, and nothing I have said casts doubt on the proposition that the doing of a positive act with the intention of ending life is and remains murder.'[13]

Tony Bland was a victim of the Hillesborough football stadium disaster, and was in a persistent vegetative state (PVS). There was an application to court to decide whether it was lawful for artificial feeding to be discontinued. The House of Lords held that there was no duty to keep him alive in those circumstances, and that artificial feeding could be discontinued and he could be allowed to die. A practice direction[14] was issued to guide professionals and lawyers in comparable PVS cases, and a declaration of the court is required before artificial feeding can be withdrawn in patients in PVS.

Because of the current uncertainties and variations in practice, the British Medical Association (BMA) issued a consultation paper on withdrawing and withholding treatment in order to develop a clearer legal framework.[15] The BMA has now issued guidance on withholding and withdrawing treatment.[16]

Living wills/advance refusal or directive

A mentally competent person can decide in advance that at a subsequent time he or she would not wish to receive treatment. At present we do not have any statutory provision (i.e. Act of Parliament) recognising living wills. However, they would be recognised by common law (i.e. judge-made law, or case law). This was stated by the House of Lords in the Tony Bland case.[17] Living wills (also known as advance refusals or advance directives) are designed to convey the wishes of an adult, when mentally competent, to cover a future occasion when mental competence is lacking. The BMA has published a Code of Practice for its members on advance statements about medical treatment.[18] It gives guidance on the law in relation to consent to medical treatment and advance statements, and advice on the drafting and contents of an advance statement. It emphasises that there must be no pressure on patients. It also gives guidance on determining the patient's capacity to make decisions. The responsibility for storing an advance directive is on the individual, but it is suggested that a copy should be given to the general practitioner. Finally, a check-list is provided for making an advance directive (this is shown in Box 17.4).

Box 17.4:   British Medical Association check-list for writing an advance statement

In drawing up an advance statement you must ensure, as a minimum, that the following information is included.

- Full name.
- Address.
- Name and address of general practitioner.
- Whether advice was sought from health professionals.
- Signature.
- Date drafted and reviewed.
- Witness signature.
- A clear statement of your wishes (either general or specific).
- The name, address and telephone number of your nominated person, if you have one.

Letting die: the mentally incompetent adult; acting in the best interests under Re F principle; Law Commission proposals – and who decides?

At present there is a vacuum in the law in that no person has the right to make decisions on behalf of the mentally incompetent adult. Once the patient is considered to be mentally incompetent, the House of Lords has declared that health professionals should act in the best interests of that individual, following the Bolam test.[19] Health professionals can therefore, in that person's best interests, overrule any refusal. It is important that the fact of the mental incompetence is determined, and there are considerable advantages if a person outside the multidisciplinary team can determine the competence of the patient. Competence must be decided in the light of the decision to be made. In the case of MB, the Court of Appeal held that suffering from needle phobia rendered a pregnant woman mentally incompetent, and therefore a Caesarean section could be carried out in her best interests without her consent.

Filling the vacuum

The present situation is unsatisfactory, and a strong case has been made by the Law Commission[20] for legislation to be enacted which would establish a statutory framework for decisions to be made on behalf of the mentally incompetent adult. The Lord

Chancellor has issued a consultation document,[21] and the Government has published its proposals for a statutory framework for decision making.[22] Until these proposals are enacted professionals must act in the best interests of the mentally incompetent adult because of the House of Lords ruling in the case of Re F.

Not For Resuscitation instructions

It follows from what has been said that a competent adult patient can request that there should be no resuscitation. This request can be made either by means of an advance refusal or by refusing resuscitation when admitted for that particular course of treatment. However, if the patient is mentally incompetent and has made no advance refusal, then the professional has a duty to take all reasonable care of the patient, and in certain cases this may involve providing resuscitation. If the prognosis is good, and there is no valid refusal of treatment by the patient, failure to resuscitate could in certain circumstances be a criminal act. However, if the clinician is of the view that the prognosis is extremely poor, a Not For Resuscitation (NFR) or Do Not Resuscitate (DNR) instruction is valid. Difficulties can arise if such instructions are not given in writing by doctors to nursing staff, or if nurses have not had an input into the decision-making and are unaware of or disagree with the basis of the NFR/DNR instruction. A report has been issued by the Royal College of Nursing[23] that sets out the moral and legal issues and strongly endorses the involvement of the healthcare professional team as well as the patient, their relatives and friends.[24] The views of relatives may be relevant to the decision, and certainly any evidence they can give of the patient's wishes will be important, but the relatives do not have the right in law to give or withhold consent to resuscitation.

Record-keeping

Inevitably, if there is any criticism of the care and treatment of the patient, the records become the focus of evidence. However, records should not be seen as part of defensive practice. Maintaining high standards of record-keeping is part of the professional duty of care owed to the patient. One test for determining the standard of record-keeping is to imagine a situation in which a professional looking after certain patients was removed from the workplace without notice and without being able to give messages to their colleagues. Could their colleagues take over responsibility for those patients and provide continuity of care for them based on the records kept by the missing professional?

If the records pass this test, then they are likely to be of sufficient standard to protect the professional in the event of any litigation, complaint or other proceedings. In other words, the prime reason for ensuring high standards of record-keeping is the care of the patient, but high standards will also provide protection for professionals when their care is subject to scrutiny. Regular audit of record-keeping standards by colleagues in a constructive way is essential to maintaining and improving standards.

Statements

In the event of a patient dying unexpectedly or in certain specified circumstances (e.g. in prison or whilst detained under the Mental Health Act), the death would be reported to the coroner, who may decide to hold an inquest. The coroner might order a post-mortem and then request statements from those who were involved in the care of the patient. It is advisable to obtain senior management or legal advice when preparing a statement. The statement may be used in subsequent criminal or civil proceedings, and could be used in disciplinary or professional conduct proceedings.

Statutory framework for the provision of healthcare

The impact of the White Paper and the Health Services Act 1999

The Health Services Act 1999 has implemented the recommendations made in the White Paper.[25] Primary care groups established in England (and local health groups in Wales) commission health services from the providers. GP fundholding was abolished, and the internal market in healthcare ended. The Government is hoping that these new organisations will facilitate the shift of the emphasis from secondary to primary care. Eventually, some of these primary care groups will achieve trust status and could possibly become responsible for the provision of community health services as well as primary care. In addition, the introduction of the concept of 'Clinical Governance', implemented through a statutory duty to monitor and improve the quality of healthcare, should ensure that standards of quality improve. New institutions such as the National Institute of Clinical Excellence (NICE), the Commission for Health Improvement (CHImp) and National Standards Frameworks should lead to the dissemination of good practice and research findings on pain management. Hospitals and community providers are expected to provide clinically effective research-based treatments and care. A national framework for palliative care services would lead to national standards, which patients could use to criticise local provision and professionals could use to justify additional resources and higher standards. In future, the Bolam test may require that care is provided according to protocols, guidelines or procedures published by NICE or CHImp.

Conclusion

There will always be pressure for professionals to assist patients in ending their lives. Often the demands result from fear of pain or from a low standard of palliative care, so that patients may feel that their only respite would be assisted suicide. It is a challenge to professionals providing palliative care to ensure that patients are able to secure a dignified, pain-free death, while at the same time recognising that the law does not permit any person to take any positive action to cause the death of another.

Further reading is recommended for those who wish to study the legal and ethical issues in more detail.

References

1   Bolam v. Friern Hospital Management Committe (1957) 2 *All ER* 118.

2   Bolitho v. City and Hackney Health Authority (1997) 3 *WLR* 1151.

3   R v. Adomako' House of Lords (1994) *The Times Law Report*. 4 July.

4   Coke, 3 Co Inst 47 (Law Report Series).

5   Wilkinson P (1998) Daughter walks free over 'mercy killing'. *The Times*. 30 June.

6   R v. Cox (1992) *The Times*. 22 September.

7   Bedford S (1961) *The Best We Can Do*. Penguin, Harmondsworth.

8   Wilkins E (1997) Dying woman granted wish for dignified death. *The Times*. 29 October.

9   Re T (1992) 4 *All ER* 649.

10 In re M B (Caesarian section) (1997) *The Times Law Report*. 18 April.

11 Rachels J (ed) (1971) *Moral Problems*. Harper and Row, New York.

12 Harris J (1985) *The Value of Life*. Routledge and Kegan Paul, London.

13 Airedale NHS Trust v. Bland House of Lords (1993) 1 *All ER* 821.

14 Practice Note (Vegetative State) (1996) 2 *FLR* 375.

15 BMA Medical Ethics Committee (1998) *BMA Withdrawing and Withholding Treatment: a Consultation Paper*. British Medical Association, London.

16 British Medical Association (1999) *Withholding and Withdrawing Life-prolonging Medical Treatment*. BMA, London.

17 Airedale NHS Trust v. Bland House of Lords (1993) 1 *All ER* 821.

18 British Medical Association (1995) *Advance Statements about Medical Treatment: Code of Practice*. British Medical Association, London.

19   F v. Berkshire HA (1989) **2** *All ER* 545.

20   Law Commission (1995) *Mental Incapacity Report No. 231*. HMSO, London.

21   Lord Chancellor's Office (1997) *Lord Chancellor – Who Decides?*

22   Lord Chancellor's Office (1999) *Making Decisions*. The Stationery Office, London.

23   Royal College of Nursing (1992) *Resuscitation: Right or Wrong? The Moral and Legal Issues Faced by Health Care Professionals.*

24   Dimond B (1992) Not for resuscitative treatment. *Br J Nursing.* **1**: 93–4.

25   Department of Health (1997) *The New NHS: Modern, Dependable*. The Stationery Office, London.

To learn more

Dimond BC (1995) *Legal Aspects of Nursing* (2e). Prentice-Hall, Hemel Hempstead.

Dimond BC (1997) *Legal Aspects of Care in the Community*. Macmillan Press, London.

Dimond BC (1998) *Patient's Rights, Responsibilities and the Nurse* (2e). Central Health Studies Quay Publishing, Salisbury.

Greaves D and Upton H (eds) (1996) *The Right to Die*. Euthanasia and Advanced Directives, Avebury.

Kennedy I and Grubb A (1994) *Medical Law. Text and Materials* (2e). Butterworths, London.

McHale J and Fox H (1997) *Health Care Law. Text and Materials*. Sweet and Maxwell, London.

McHale J, Tingle J and Peysner J (1998) *Law and Nursing*. Butterworth-Heinemann, Oxford.

Mason JK and McCall Smith RA (1994) *Law and Medical Ethics* (4e). Butterworths, London.

Appendix: Useful contacts

Alzheimer's Disease Society
Gordon House
10 Greencoat Place
London
SW1P 1PH

Tel: 020 7306 0606

This society provides advice and support for carers and day and home care.

Bereavement Research Forum
Bereavement Care
The Linda Machin Centre Rooms
The Dudson Centre
Hope Street
Hanley
Stoke-on-Trent
ST1 5DD

Tel: 01782 683 155

A multiprofessional group that aims to facilitate networking between bereavement researchers.

Breast Cancer Care
Kiln House
210 New Kings Road
London
SW6 4NZ

Nationwide Freeline: 0500 245 345
(Monday to Friday, 10 a.m. to 7 p.m.)

Offers practical advice, information and support to women concerned about breast cancer. Its services include a wide range of booklets, leaflets and audiotapes, a prosthesis-fitting service and one-to-one emotional support from volunteers who have themselves experienced breast cancer. Breast Cancer Care aims to help anyone who needs its services – not only women with breast cancer or other breast-related problems, but also their families, partners and friends, women who are worried about their breast health, members of the general public who need information, doctors, nurses and other health professionals, and the media.

Bristol Cancer Help Centre
Grove House
Cornwallis Grove
Bristol
BC8 4PG

Helpline: 0117 980 9505

This centre offers a healing programme that deals with the whole person and is complementary to medical treatment. People affected by cancer are offered relaxation, healing, visualisation, counselling, nutrition therapy, meditation, music and art therapy. The centre runs one-day courses, a residential week and follow-up days. There are also educational programmes for health professionals. A charge is made for services, but discretionary bursaries are available.

Cancerlink
11–21 Northdown Street
London
N1 9BN

Freephone Cancer Information Helpline: 0800 132 905 (Textphone available)
Freephone Asian Cancer Information Helpline: 0800 590 415

Provides emotional support and information in response to telephone enquiries and letters on all aspects of cancer, from people with cancer, their families, friends and professionals working with them. It is a resource to over 600 cancer support and self-help groups throughout the UK, and helps people who are setting up new groups. Free publications and audiotapes in seven languages are available.

CANCERBACUP
3 Bath Place
Rivington Street
London
EC2A 3JR

Freephone Cancer Information Service: 0800 181199
(Monday to Friday, 9 a.m. to 7 p.m.)
Cancer Counselling Service London: 020 7696 9000
(Monday to Friday, 9 a.m. to 5.30 p.m.)

Cancer Counselling Service Glasgow: 0141 553 1553
(Monday to Friday, 9 a.m. to 5.30 p.m.)
Textphone available; BACUP website:
www.cancerbacup.org.uk

This organisation helps people with cancer, their families and friends live with cancer. Specialist cancer nurses provide information, emotional support and practical advice by telephone and letter. A range of free publications and a magazine are available. Professional counsellors provide face-to-face counselling free of charge and in confidence in London and Glasgow.

Carers National Association
20–25 Glasshouse Yard
London
EC1A 4JS

Carer line: 0345 573 369
(Monday to Friday, 10 a.m. to 12 noon and 2 p.m. to 4 p.m.)

Offers information and support to people caring for family and friends. The Association has over 100 branches all over the UK which are run by carers and can refer carers to local sources of help and support. The Association also has offices in Northern Ireland, Scotland and Wales, and lobbies Government, both local and national, on behalf of carers. It offers a range of free leaflets and information sheets.

Compassionate Friends
53 North Street
Bristol
BS3 1EN

Tel: 0117 953 9639

A support group for parents who have lost a child.

CRUSE Bereavement Care
Cruse House
126 Sheen Road
Richmond
Surrey
TW9 1UR

Tel: 020 8332 7227

A support group for widows and widowers.

Hospice Information Service
St Christopher's Hospice
51–59 Lawrie Park Road
Sydenham
London
SE26 6DZ

Tel: 020 8778 9252

The Hospice Information Service publishes a directory of hospice and palliative care services which provides details of hospices, home-care teams and hospital-support teams in the UK and the Republic of Ireland. For copies of the directory or details of local services, please send a large SAE with three first-class stamps, or telephone.

Huntington's Disease Association
108 Battersea High Street
London
SW11 3HP

Tel: 020 7223 7000

Institute for Complementary Medicine
PO Box 194
London
SE16 1QZ

Tel: 020 7237 5165

The Institute supplies information on qualified and complementary practitioners, complementary teaching institutions and complementary medicine, generally for use by the media. Enquirers are asked to supply an SAE and two loose stamps. The ICM will not diagnose either on the telephone or by letter. It administers the national British Register of Complementary Practitioners, and its members are qualified, fully insured and follow a Code of Conduct.

Institute of Family Therapy
24–32 Stephenson Way
London
NW1 2HX

Tel: 020 7391 9150

A registered charity that provides a comprehensive service to families and couples who are experiencing difficulty, including copying with family illness, loss and bereavement. Its approach is based on helping people to explore their difficulties in terms of their family and other close relationships. Families/couples are asked to contribute according to a sliding scale of fees based on income.

Let's Face It
14 Fallowfield
Yateley
Hampshire
GU46 6LW

Tel: 01252 879 630

A contact point for people of any age coping with facial disfigurement. Provides a link for people with similar experiences, telephone and letter contact, meeting for self-help or social contact.

Macmillan Cancer Relief
Anchor House
15–19 Britten Street
London
SW3 3TZ

Tel: 020 7351 7811
Macmillan information line: 0845 601 6161
(Monday to Friday, 9.30 a.m. to 4.30 p.m.)

A national charity working to improve the treatment and care of people with cancer and their families from the point of diagnosis. Specialist Macmillan nurses, Macmillan doctors, buildings for cancer treatment and care, grants for patients in financial difficulty. Information on Macmillan services and activities available through national Macmillan Information Line. Applications for patients' grants through Macmillan nurses, community nurses, health and social workers and local voluntary organisations.

Marie Curie Cancer Care
28 Belgrave Square
London
SW1X 8QG

Tel: 020 7235 3325

A cancer care charity that provides practical hands-on nursing care at home and specialist multidisciplinary care through its 11 Marie Curie Centres. Both services are available throughout the UK and are assessed through the local district nursing service and GPs/consultants respectively. Both services are free of charge to patients.

Motor Neurone Disease Association
PO Box 246
Northampton
NN1 2PR

Tel: 01604 250 505
Helpline: 0345 626 262

Provides advice and information for people with motor neurone disease, their carers and professionals.

Multiple Sclerosis Society
25 Effie Road
Fulham
London
SW6 1EE

Tel: 020 7610 7171
Helpline: 020 7371 8000

Provides information for people with MS and their families and carers.

National Association of Bereavement Services
20 Norton Folgate
London
E1 6DB

Tel: 020 7247 1080

A membership and support organisation for bereavement services within the UK.

Parkinson's Disease Society
22 Upper Woburn Place
London
WC1H 0RA

Tel: 020 7383 3513
Helpline: 020 7388 5798

Provides welfare information, education and services for people with Parkinson's disease, their families and professionals.

Stroke Association
Stroke House
123–127 Whitecross Street
London EC1Y 8JJ
Tel: 020 7490 7999

Provides advice, information, community services and welfare grants. Also runs local stroke clubs for support.

Index

accountability in pain management 236–8
Activities of Living Model 92
acupuncture 174
Adams, Dr Bodkin 240–1
admission
  hospice, criteria
    day unit 171–2
    in-patient service 161–3
  hospital 193–4
advance statement 242, 243
affective disturbance, stress-related 198
alarms, syringe driver 56
alginates 100
alimentary tract, see constipation;
    gastrointestinal tract
allergy to metal (cannula) 61–3
Alzheimer's Disease Society 249
amyotrophic lateral sclerosis, see motor
    neurone disease
analgesia (pharmacological) 5–17
  compliance 5–6
  mouth pain 76
  syringe drivers for 62
  WHO three-step ladder 6
antidepressants 50
anti-emetics 29
  in syringe drivers 62
antifungals, thrush 76
anti-inflammatory drugs, bone pain 13–14
antipsychotics in confusion 49
anxiety (and fear)
  in motor neurone disease
    family 228
    patient 227–8
  pain increase with 18
anxiolytics (incl. benzodiazepines)
  confusion 49
  pain control via 18
  in syringe drivers 62

terminal restlessness 108–10
aromatherapy 174
ascites 51
aspirin, bone pain 14
assessment/evaluation
  in-patient service 166
  in integrated care pathway, initial 181,
    182
  patient
    fungating wounds 92–8
    hospice day unit suitability 172
    in motor neurone disease 225–30
    oedema 82–3
    oral 69–70, 71
    pain, see pain
    terminal restlessness 106–7
audit, in-patient service 166
autonomy, patient 241
aversion therapy, nausea/vomiting 29

bad news, breaking 156
Barriers to Research Utilisation Scale 214
behaviour, stress-related 198
behaviour therapy, nausea/vomiting 29
Belbin Self-Perception Inventory 211
benzodiazepines, see anxiolytics
bereavement 137–47
  in-patient services 165
  motor neurone disease 232
  useful contacts 254
Bereavement Research Forum 249
bicarbonate, mouth cleansing 73
bisphosphonates
  bone pain 14
  hypercalcaemia 45
Bland, Tony 242
body image and fungating wounds 94–5
Bolam test 237, 243, 245
bone pain, opioid-unresponsive 13–14

Bonjela   76
bowel obstruction   38–43
    syringe drivers delivering drugs in   62
    see also constipation; gastrointestinal tract
brachial plexus neuropathy   87
breaking bad news   156
Breast Cancer Care   249
breathing and fungating wounds   93
Breathing Space Kit   231
breathlessness, see dyspnoea
Bristol Cancer Help Centre   250
British Medical Association and withdrawing/
    withholding of treatment   242
bulking agents   37
burnout   198–9
Buscopan in syringe drivers   62
butyrophenones, see haloperidol

Calman/Hine report   154
cancer
    advanced, lymphoedema, see lymphoedema
    bone pain (with metastases), opioid-
        unresponsive   13–14
    fungating wounds, see wounds
    useful contacts   249–50, 251–2
CANCERBACUP   250
Cancerlink   250
candidiasis, oral (thrush)   76
    assessment   71
cannula, metal allergy   61–3
capillary filtration rate and oedema   81–2
care
    right to refuse   241
    standard of, in pain management   236,
        237
carers   119–25
    defining   119–20
    feelings/emotions   120–1, 195, 199
    needs   121–3
    professional, see professional carers
    see also family/relatives
Carers National Association   251
causation   237
change   212–13
    communicating   193
    management of   212–13

chaplain
    day unit   175
    in-patient unit   165
charcoal, activated   100
children and motor neurone disease patients
    228–9
chiropody   165
chlorhexidine   73
choline salicylate gel   76
circulation list   193
civil liability and pain management   236
cleansing agents, oral   73
clinical nurse specialist, see specialist nurse
cognitive factors in work stress
    as protective factors   202
    as sequelae   198
cognitive interventions, terminal restlessness
    108
collaboration, in-patient unit   163–4
Commission for Health Improvement
    (CHImp)   245
communication (by patient), assessment
    in motor neurone disease   227
        family and   228
    non-verbal communication   71
communication (by professionals to other
    professionals and patient/family)   189–
    96, 213–14
    to patient (specifically)
        fungating wounds   92–3
        and relatives and specialist nurses in in-
            patient setting   164–5
        terminal restlessness and   112–13
    see also information
community professional   207–19
    caring for   207–19
    multifaceted role   208–9
Compassionate Friends   251
complementary treatment
    hospice day unit   174
    hospice in-patient   165
    nausea/vomiting   29
    useful contacts   250
confusion   46–50
    acute confusional state, see delirium
consent and the law   241

constipation 35–43
  with morphine 8
  see also bowel obstruction
continuous subcutaneous infusion 55–65
coping with stress 203
coroner requesting statements 245
Corsodyl 73
corticosteroids, see steroids
cost and communication issues 195
counselling
  in-patient service 165
  referral for 166
counter-transference 145
courses, nurse specialist 155
Cox, Dr Nigel 240
creative activities
  day unit 174
  in-patient unit 165
CRUSE Bereavement Care 251
cyclizine 29
  in syringe drivers 62

day hospice care 169–76
  motor neurone disease 230
death, sudden, bereavement problems 143
debriefing, team 133
delirium 105–6
  restlessness with 110–11
dentition
  assessment 71
  plaque 68–9, 72
dentures
  assessment 71
  care 73–4
depersonalisation, professionals 199
depression 50
dexamethasone
  bowel obstruction 40
  spinal cord compression 45
  in syringe drivers 62
diamorphine (heroin) 10
  conversion from fentanyl patch to 11–12
  converting from morphine to 10
  in motor neurone disease 231
  in syringe drivers 62
diazepam

in pain control 18
  in terminal restlessness 109–10
diclofenac, bone pain 14
diet, see nutrition
discharge (from care) 194
  from in-patient unit, day care following
    175
distress, dealing with 156
diversional activities
  day unit 174
  fungating wounds 96
  in-patient unit 165
Do Not Resuscitate instructions 244
documentation, see record-keeping
domperidone 29
dressings 100
drinking, see nutrition
drowsiness, see sedation
drugs
  adverse effects
    skin irritation 63
    xerostomia 75
  analgesic, see analgesia
  anti-emetic 29
  in bowel obstruction and constipation 37,
    40–1
  in confusion 49
  in depression 50
  in flushing/sweating 52
  in motor neurone disease 231–2
  in pruritus 51
  in syringe drivers 61, 62
  in terminal restlessness 108–11
  see also specific drugs
dry mouth 74–5
duty of care and accountability in pain
  management 236–8
dying and wound care 95
dysphagia in motor neurone disease 226–7
dyspnoea (breathlessness) 30–4
  in motor neurone disease 226, 231

eating, see nutrition
economic aspects, see financial aspects
education and training (in palliative care)
  214–15

integrated care pathways and   185
   nurse specialist   155
   see also teaching
elimination of waste, fungating wounds and
   93
emesis, *see* vomiting and nausea
emotions/feelings
   carers (in general incl. family/relatives)
     120–1
   patients, causing restlessness   111–12
   professionals (incl. nurses)   195, 199
     in coping with stress   203
     negative feelings relating to
       bereavement   145
employee liability   238
enemas   37
euthanasia   239
   trials concerning   240–1
evaluation, *see* assessment

facial disfigurement   94
   useful contacts   249
faecal incontinence and fungating wounds
   93
faecal softeners   37
family/relatives
   bereavement, *see* bereavement
   external family system   210
   hospice day care and   171
   motor neurone disease and   228–9
   mouthcare and   70
   pain assessment and   19
   relationships, *see* relationships
   respite care   162–3
   spiritual issues   130
   support, *see* support
   terminal restlessness and   108, 112, 113
   see also carers
fatigue, case management   42–6
fear, *see* anxiety
feelings, *see* emotions
fentanyl   10–12
   lozenge   12
   transdermal patch   9, 10–12
fever in wound infection   93
film dressings   100

financial/economic aspects of motor neurone
   disease   228
fluconazole, thrush   76
fluid accumulation, *see* oedema
flurbiprofen, bone pain   14
flushes   51–2
foam dressings   100
foam sticks   72
friendship vs therapeutic relationship   145

gastrointestinal tract, nausea/vomiting
   relating to   25
   see also constipation
gingiva, *see* gums
glycerine and lemon swabs   73
glycerine of thymol   73
God   131
granisetron   29
gums/gingiva, assessment   71

haloperidol
   confusion   49
   nausea/vomiting   29
   in syringe drivers   62
   terminal restlessness   110
health professionals, *see* professional carers
Health Services Act (1999)   245
heroin, *see* diamorphine
hiccups   50–1
homicide, *see* murder
hope, encouraging   128
hospice
   community nurse working within   208–9
   day unit, *see* day hospice care
   in-patient unit, *see* in-patient unit
   structure   208–9
Hospice Information Service   252
Huntington's Disease Association   252
hydrocolloids sheets   100
hydromorphone   9
hydropolymer dressings   100
hyoscine butylbromide in syringe drivers   62
hyoscine hydrochloride
   motor neurone disease   232
   in syringe drivers   62
hypercalcaemia   43–4, 45

hypothermia and wound healing 93
hypoxia, tissue, fungating wounds 90

ibuprofen, bone pain 14
incontinence and fungating wounds 93
infection
    fungal, *see* candidiasis
    wound, pyrexia in 93
information
    for health/social care professionals,
        communicating 192–3, 194
        on discharge 194
    for patient, on discharge 194
    see also communication
in-patient unit, hospice 161–8
    day care following discharge from 175
    motor neurone disease 230
Institute for Complementary Medicine 252
Institute of Family Therapy 252
integrated care pathways 179–86
    associated guidelines 183–4
    defining 180
    implementing 182–3
    information generated from, and feedback
        loop 184
    initiating 180
    variations from pathway 184
    writing 181–2
intestine, *see* bowel obstruction; constipation;
    gastrointestinal tract
itching (pruritus) 51

job-related stress 199–202

ketorolac
    bone pain 14
    in syringe drivers 62

law 235–47
Law Commission proposals 243–4
laxatives 37
leadership 211–12
legal issues 235–47
lemon and glycerine swabs 73
Let's Face It 253
levomepromazine (methotrimeprazine)

confusion 49
nausea/vomiting 29
in syringe drivers 62
terminal restlessness 109, 110
liability
    as employee 238
    professional 238
    vicarious 237–8
lifestyle management, community nurses
    216
limb
    function/movement, nerve compression
        affecting 86–7
    mobilisation 94
lips, assessment 71
listening
    bereaved persons 144
    spirituality and 130
Liverpool Care Pathway 181, 182
living wills 242
loss
    by bereaved relatives 137–8
        nature 143
    concept of 137–8
    by palliative care workers, accumulated
        201–2
lymphatic system
    drainage, stimulating 85
    reduced transport capacity 82
lymphoedema 81–8, 165
    assessment 82–3
    complications 86–7
    management 84–5
lymphorrhoea 86

Macmillan Cancer Relief 253
malignant tumours, *see* cancer
malodour, fungating wounds 95, 97–8
management issues 207–19
manslaughter 238–9
    euthanasia and 239
Marie Curie Cancer Care 253
martyr syndrome 146
massage
    self-, lymph drainage stimulated via 85
    shiatsu, hospice day unit 174

terminal restlessness 108
mental competence and the law 241–2
mental incompetence and the law 243
metal (cannula), allergy 61–3
methadone 9
methotrimeprazine, *see* levomepromazine
metoclopramide 29
    in syringe drivers 62
midazolam
    confusion 49
    motor neurone disease 232
    in syringe drivers 62
    terminal restlessness 108–9
mood (affective) disturbance, stress-related
        198
Morcap 9
morphine 7–8
    dose increases 8
    fear of dependency 5–6
    oral 7
        conversion to diamorphine 10
        conversion to fentanyl patch 11
        quick-release, fentanyl patches and 11
    side-effects 8–9
morphine sulphate tablet 7, 7–8
motor neurone disease 223–34
    bereavement 233
    diagnosis 223–5
    legal issues 241
    progression 225–30
    terminal stages 230–2
Motor Neurone Disease Association 254
mourning 139
mouth care (oral problems) 67–79
    good, definition and aim 68–9
    poor
        causes 69
        effects 68
    regime 72
    tools and agents 72–3
mouthwashes 73
MS16^A syringe driver
    differences from MS26 55, 56, 57
    flow rate calculation 63
    general description/features 55, 57
    setting up 59

requirements 59
MS26 syringe driver
    boost facility 60–1
    differences from MS16^A 55, 56, 57
    flow rate calculation 63
    general description/features 55, 58
    setting up 59
    requirements 59
MST 7, 7–8
MST suspension 7, 9
mucosa/mucous membranes, oral 69
    assessment 71
Multiple Sclerosis Society 254
murder 238–41
    defined 239
MXL 9

National Association of Bereavement
        Services 254
National Institute of Clinical Excellence
        (NICE) 245
nausea, *see* vomiting and nausea
needs, carers 121–3
negligence and pain management 236, 237
neoplasms, malignant, *see* cancer
nerve compression, limb function affected by
        86–7
nerve pain, opioid-unresponsive 14–15
neuroleptics in confusion 49
neurological patient, special needs 223–34
night, waking with pain 8
non-steroidal anti-inflammatory drugs, bone
        pain 13–14
Not For Resuscitation instructions 244
NSAIDs, bone pain 13–14
nutrition (diet incl. eating and drinking)
    fungating wounds 93
    in-patient service 165
nystatin, thrush 76

occupational therapy
    day unit 174–5
    in-patient unit 165
octreotide (somatostatin analogue) 29, 41
    in syringe drivers 62
odour, fungating wounds 95, 97–8

oedema 81–8
  assessment 82–3
  causes 81–2
  complications 86–7
  lymphatic, *see* lymphoedema
  management 84–5
ondansetron 29
  in syringe drivers 62
opioids 7–15
  compliance 5–6
  pain unresponsive to 13–15, 16
  prescribing considerations 10
  rotation 12–13
  side-effects 8–9, 10, 12, 13
  strong 6, 7–13
    long-acting 9–10
  weak 6
Orabase cream 76
oral health
  assessment 69–70, 71
  care, *see* mouth care
  common problems 74–7
Oramorph 7, 8
outcomes of care (in integrated care
    pathways) 181–2
oxycodone 9

pain (physical)
  assessment 3–4, 19, 71
    in motor neurone disease 226
  bone 13–14
  breakthrough 7, 11
    at night 8
  control/management 5–22
    aims 4
    duty of care and accountability 236–8
    non-pharmacological 5, 17–19
    pharmacological, *see* analgesia
    simple measures 5
  nerve 14–15
  opioid-unresponsive 13–15, 16
  oral 71, 76
  patient's awareness/expectations 4–5
  rapidly increasing 5
  visceral 17
  wound

  assessment 98
  management 99
pain (psychological), carer 120–5
Parkinson's Disease Society 254
peer group support, day care 171
persistent vegetative state 242
person/environment fit model of stress 199,
    200
personality and work stress 202
phenothiazines, *see* levomepromazine;
    thioridazine
photography, wound 97
physical examination, lymphoedema 83
physiotherapy, day unit 174
pineapple chunks 77
plaque, dental 68–9, 72
podiatry (chiropody) 165
position of patient in motor neurone disease,
    comfortable 226
Post-Registration Education and Practice
    report 154
primary healthcare team 153
  hospice day unit referral and 171
problem-focused strategies of coping with
    stress 203
professional carers (health and social care)
    caring for 207–19
  communication between 189–96
  emotions, *see* emotions
  hospice day unit 173–5
  in motor neurone disease terminal stages
    231
  specialist, *see* specialist nurses; specialist
    professionals
  spiritual issues 131
  stress, *see* stress
  see also team
professional liability 238
prostaglandin synthesis inhibitors, bone
    pain 13–14
pruritus 51
psychiatrist, referral to 166
psychological dimensions/issues
  fungating wounds 92–3, 95
  in lymphoedema, psychological
    assessment 83

psychological strategies
  fungating wounds 96
  pain control 18
  terminal restlessness 111–12
psychosocial assessment, lymphoedema 83
pyrexia in wound infection 93

rattle, terminal 51
record-keeping/documentation
  law and 245
  of wound assessment 98
referral
  to hospice day unit 169–71
  to hospice in-patient unit 161–3
  to psychiatrist or counsellor 166
  to specialist service 154–7
reflexology 174
refusal of care
  advance statement 242
  mental incompetence and 243
  right to refuse 241
Reiki healing 174
relationships
  family 132
    ambivalent, bereavement and 142
  nurse–bereaved person 145
  professional team 132–3
    stress and 201
relatives, *see* family
relaxation in pain control 18
religion, *see* spirituality
research findings, adopting 214–15
respite care 162–3
restlessness, terminal 105–16
resuscitate, failure to 244
right to refuse care 241
risk factors
  family bereavement problems 142–3
  in professionals
    community nurses 210
    for stress 199–203

salicylate, mouth ulcer 76
saline mouthwashes 73
saliva 69
  assessment 71

SCARED syndrome 94–5
sedation/drowsiness
  family and 112
  with morphine 7, 8
self-help, bereavement 144
Self-Perception Inventory, Belbin's 211
semi-permeable film membranes 100
Sevredol 7
sexuality
  fungating wounds and 94–5
  motor neurone disease and 228
shiatsu massage 174
silences in conversation 133
skin
  fungating wound surrounds, assessment
    97–8
  irritation, drugs causing 63
  in lymphoedema, care of problems relating
    to 84, 86
sleeping and wound care 96
smell, fungating wounds 95, 97–8
social isolation, the bereaved 142
social support strategies of coping with
    stress 203
social workers, day unit 175
  see also professional carers
sodium bicarbonate, mouth cleansing 73
softeners, faecal 37
somatostatin analogue, *see* octreotide
specialist nurses 151–60
  referral/intervention/outcome 154–7
  role boundaries 152–3
  role definition 153–4
  role transition 154
specialist professionals in in-patient services
    165–6
speech assessment in motor neurone disease
    226
speech therapy 165
spinal cord compression 44, 45
spirituality (incl. religion) 127–35
  day unit 175
  in-patient unit 165
  motor neurone disease and 229–30
  wound care and 96
staff, *see* professional carers

standard of care in pain management 236, 237
statements requested by coroner 245
statutory framework for healthcare provision 245
steroids
    pain control and 15–17
    in syringe drivers 62
    see also dexamethasone
stimulant laxatives 37
stomatitis, denture 73–4
stress
    bereaved persons 143
    professionals 197–206
        community nurses 210, 215–16
Stroke Association 254
strontium-89, bone pain 14
subcutaneous infusion 55–65
    continuous 55–65
    diamorphine 10
        conversion from fentanyl patch to 11–12
    in terminal restlessness 108–9
sucralfate, mouth ulcers 76
sudden death, bereavement problems 143
suffering, carer 120–35
suicide and the law 236, 237, 240
superior vena cava obstruction 34
supervision 133
support 249–54
    carers (in general) 123–4
    family 250–1
        in bereavement 144, 145, 254
        hospices 162–3, 164, 165
        in motor neurone disease 228–9
        terminal restlessness and 112
    patient, hospice day units and 171
    professionals (incl. nurses) 146
        community nurses 215–16
        support groups 146, 203
    useful contacts 249–54
surgery, constipation 40
swallowing, assessment 71
    in motor neurone disease 226–7
sweats 51–2
swelling, fluid causing, *see* oedema

symptoms
    control 23–53
        general principles 24–5
        in lymphoedema 85
        pain, *see* pain
    in motor neurone disease, assessment 225–7
    prevalence 23
syringe (in syringe drivers) 61
syringe drivers 55–65
    boost facility 60–1
    flow rate calculation 63
    general description/properties/characteristics 55–6
    how to use 56–8
    indications 58–9
    monitoring of patient's condition with 63–4
    setting up 59–60
        requirements for 59

taste, assessment 71
teaching, nurse specialist 156
    see also education
teams (and teamwork) 130
    communication, *see* communication
    community nurses and 209
    in-patient unit 163–4
    management issues 207–19
    primary healthcare team, *see* primary healthcare team
    relationships, *see* relationships
    supervision/reviewing/debriefing 133
teeth, *see* dentition
telecommunication 195–6
temperature, body, fungating wounds and 93
TENS 17
terminal rattle 51
terminal restlessness 105–16
terminal stages of motor neurone disease 230–2
thioridazine 49
thrush, *see* candidiasis
thymol, glycerine of 73
timeliness of loss 142

time-wasting and communication issues
    195
tiredness, case management 42–6
tissue with fungating wounds
    devitalised, percentage assessment 97
    hypoxia 90
tongue
    assessment 71
    furred 76–7
tooth, *see* dentition
toothbrush 72
toothpaste 72
training, *see* education; teaching
transactional leadership 211, 212
transcutaneous electrical nerve stimulation
    17
transdermal fentanyl patch, *see* fentanyl
transference 145
transformational leadership 212
truncal swelling 86
tumours, malignant, *see* cancer

UKCC 154
ulcers
    malignant, *see* wound
    mouth 76
United Kingdom Central Council for Nursing,
    Midwifery and Health Visiting 154
urinary symptoms 50
    urinary incontinence and fungating
        wounds 93

vena cava (superior) obstruction 34
vicarious liability 237–8
visceral pain 17
visualisation in pain control 18
voice, assessment 71
vomiting and nausea 25–30
    case management 25–30, 40
    drug management, *see* anti-emetics
    with morphine 8
    pathophysiology 27, 28

weakness, case management 42–6
White Paper and the Health Services Act
    (1999) 245
WHO three-step analgesic ladder 6
wills, living 242
withdrawing/withholding 242
work-related stress 199–202
World Health Organization three-step
    analgesic ladder 6
wounds, fungating (incl. malignant ulcer)
    89–104
    assessment 92–8
    epidemiology 90
    pathophysiology 90–1
    presentation/diagnosis 91–2
    treatment 93, 98–100
        aims 92
        principles 98–100

xerostomia 74–5